# Colonial American Medicine

# Colonial American

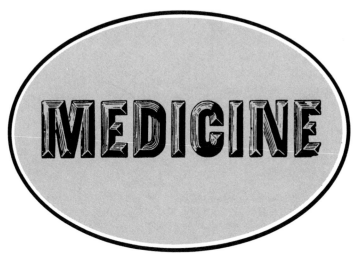

MEDICINE

## by Susan Neiburg Terkel

COLONIAL AMERICA

**FRANKLIN WATTS**

NEW YORK / CHICAGO / LONDON / TORONTO / SYDNEY

Photographs copyright ©: The M. and M. Karolik Fund, Museum of
Fine Arts, Boston: p. 12; New York Public Library, Picture Collection:
pp. 16, 27; Historical Pictures/Stock Montage: p. 19; North Wind Picture
Archives, Alfred, ME: pp. 20, 25, 32, 37, 63; Library of Congress: p. 21;
Reprinted from *The Illustrated Treasury of Medical Curiosa*, 1988, McGraw-
Hill: pp. 31 top, 35; Reprinted from *The Story of Childbirth*, 1933, Double-
day: p. 31 bottom; National Library of Medicine, Bethesda, MD: p. 44;
The Bettmann Archive: pp. 47, 53, 55, 57, 60, 71, 75, 83, 86, 89; Dittrick
Museum of Medical History/Davis and Geck: p. 78

Library of Congress Cataloging-in-Publication Data

Terkel, Susan Neiburg.
    Colonial American medicine / by Susan Neiburg Terkel.
        p.   cm.—(Colonial America)
    Includes bibliographical references and index.
    Summary: Examines the health risks in the American colonies during
the seventeenth and eighteenth centuries and looks at the
questionable, and even dangerous, treatments and remedies available
at the time.
    ISBN 0-531-12539-4
    1. Medicine—United States—History—17th century. 2. Medicine
—United States—History—18th century. [1. Medicine—History.
2. Medicine—United States—History—17th century. 3. Medicine
—United States—History—18th century.] I. Title.
R151.T43   1993
362.1'0973'09032—dc20                        92-43988   CIP   AC

# Acknowledgments

Gratitude goes to my editor, Iris Rosoff, my agent, Andrea Brown, and to John Duffy, Ph.D., an expert on colonial medicine, who carefully read over this manuscript.

Appreciation also goes to James Wilkens and Pat Jenkins, and a special thank you to my husband, Larry.

# Contents

This book is dedicated to Sue and Bert Goldberg

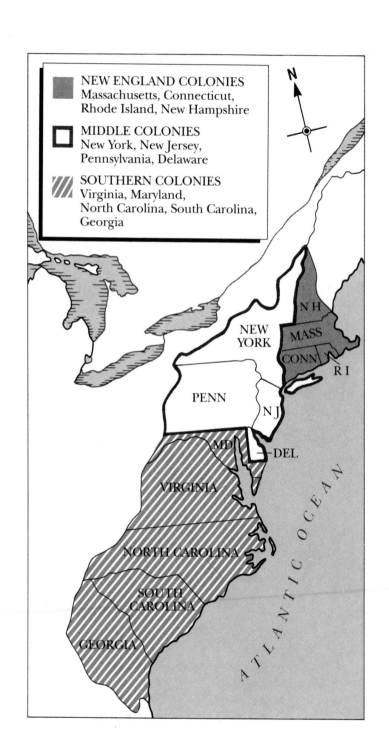

**NEW ENGLAND COLONIES**
Massachusetts, Connecticut,
Rhode Island, New Hampshire

**MIDDLE COLONIES**
New York, New Jersey,
Pennsylvania, Delaware

**SOUTHERN COLONIES**
Virginia, Maryland,
North Carolina, South Carolina,
Georgia

N

N H

NEW
YORK

MASS

CONN

R I

PENN

N J

MD

DEL

VIRGINIA

NORTH CAROLINA

SOUTH
CAROLINA

GEORGIA

ATLANTIC OCEAN

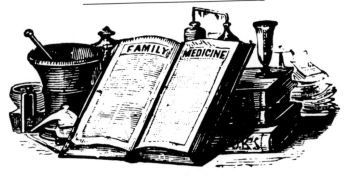

## CHAPTER ONE

# A Case History

At the close of the colonial era, on a cold, nasty day in December 1799, George Washington rode horseback across his Mount Vernon estate. Through rain and snow, he trotted and galloped. It might have been a fine ride. But soon afterward Washington took to bed with a severe cold and sore throat.

In order to reduce the vascular tension—"excess" pressure in the veins, suspected of causing his fever— Washington asked his plantation overseer to "bleed" him.[1] Using a lancet especially for the task, the overseer deftly cut open a few of Washington's veins, then collected the blood that freely flowed from them. This practice, common throughout colonial days, is known as phlebotomy.

When the illness persisted, Dr. James Craik was summoned.

Dr. Craik examined Washington and found him in a grave state. To ensure that his famous patient received the best advice, Dr. Craik consulted with Drs. Elisha Cullen Dick and Gustavus Richard Brown. The

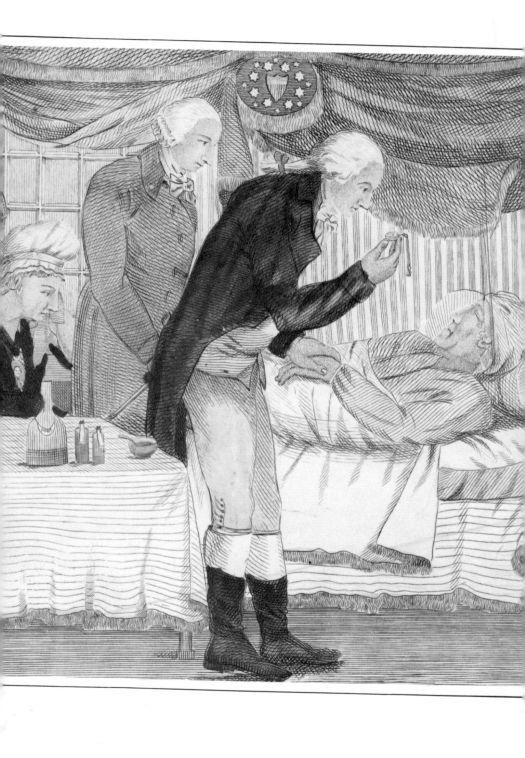

three physicians hovered over the gravely ill sixty-seven-year-old Washington, who was having difficulty breathing. What to do?

To aid his breathing, the physicians debated whether to surgically open Washington's throat with a tracheotomy, which in 1799 was dangerous. Failing to agree on such surgery, they rejected the idea and followed a different course of treatment.

A mixture of ground beetles (Spanish flies) was applied to Washington's throat, which caused blisters to form that the doctors hoped would draw out the "bad vapors." To purge his bowels, strong cathartics (medicine that causes bowel movements) were given. A poultice of vinegar and water was applied to his chest. Finally, to "reduce the tension" flowing through his veins and bring down his fever, the bloodletting was continued for several days, until 96 ounces—or one-half of Washington's total volume of blood—were drawn.

Soon George Washington slipped into a coma and died.

If medical ignorance and treatments such as bloodletting, purging, and blistering prevailed among *eminent* physicians and *notable* patients at the *end* of the colonial era, one can only imagine the state of medicine during the rest of the period. Indeed, colonial medicine was marked by ignorant theories, ineffective treatments, a scarcity of trained physicians, poor sanitation, and frightening epidemics.

Despite important discoveries like the circulation of blood, little was known about the causes of disease.

Dr. Craik and Dr. Brown try to determine the best treatment for their ailing patient, George Washington.

Without such information, medical theories remained full of grave errors, and medical treatment was rather hit and miss.

There were no laws to govern practitioners nor examinations to license them. Anyone could practice medicine, and many people did. Barbers pulled teeth and performed amputations, housewives dispensed herbal remedies and delivered babies, and businessmen, politicians, and clergy ministered to the sick. Even astrologers gave medical advice.

Treatment was often as dangerous and wretched as the disease it was supposed to help—and sometimes worse. Patients were frequently bled, induced to vomit, or purged with powerful drugs like calomel, which was later found to cause mercury poisoning.

Given how little anyone knew and how dangerous the treatments were, in many cases patients were probably better off without any reliance on the medicine of the day. One astute colonial physician, Dr. William Douglass of Boston, observed, "In general the physical practice in our colonies is so perniciously bad that excepting in surgery and in some very acute cases, it is better to let nature under a proper regimen take her course than to trust to the honesty and sagacity of the practitioner."[2]

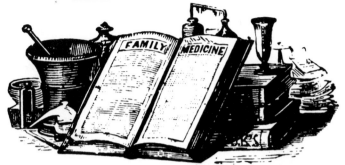

## CHAPTER TWO

# Off to a Rough Start

**M**ost settlers journeyed to the New World with courage and optimism. Almost immediately though, their high hopes—and health—were seriously tested.

For many weeks, over restless, sometimes stormy seas, they were crowded into small cabins or dark, dank holds. In these cramped, filthy, and foul-smelling quarters, diseases spread.

Lacking fresh fruit, practically everyone suffered from scurvy, which weakened their bodies and confused their minds. Rotten food—or too little food—and black, dirty, wormy water caused further hardship and often death.

"Many people whimper, sigh, and cry out pitifully for home," wrote Gottfried Mittelberger of his trip across the Atlantic, "at the thought that many hundreds of people must necessarily perish ... and be thrown into the ocean in such misery."[1]

And perish they did. Young children and birthing mothers rarely survived the passage. Dozens of others died of disease, starvation, and accidents. Some even

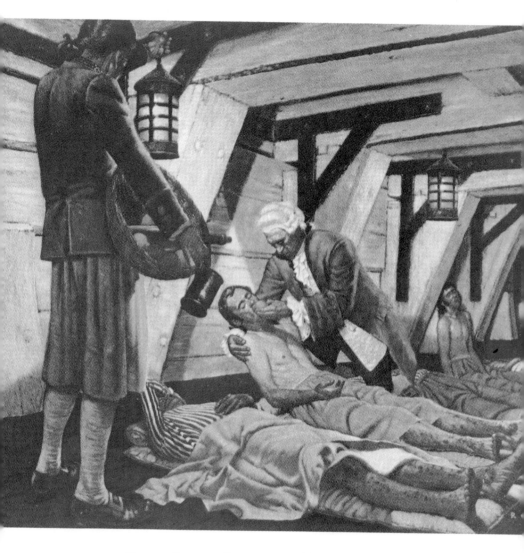

From 1600 to 1800, scurvy killed a million seamen. Here, Dr. James Lind, a surgeon in the British Royal Navy, is conducting one of many experiments to find a cure. Through such medical inquiry he learned that citrus fruits and their juices could prevent scurvy.

tumbled into the sea.[2] One Virginia-bound vessel lost over two-thirds of its passengers. Another delivered only 50 survivors out of 180 who began the sail.[3]

Upon landing, most of those who did survive the arduous passage quickly succumbed to the "cruell diseases as Swellings, Fluxes, Burning fevers, and by Warres. . . . There were never Englishmen left in a foreigne Countrey in such miserie as wee were in this new discovered Virginia."[4]

Nor did their weakened state allow the settlers to meet the challenge their new land presented. Too frail to clear ground for planting (and in some cases, too "gentlemanly") and too tired to build adequate shelter, many settlers died from starvation and exposure. "Our food was but a small can of Barlie sod in water to five men a day," wrote George Percy of the severe food shortage during his first summer in Jamestown.[5]

During the first few years, the dire situation failed to improve because the settlers had scant supplies, no crops to harvest, and they feared an Indian ambush if they ventured beyond their camp to search for food. The winter of 1609–10 in Jamestown was so bad, in fact, that colonists referred to it as "the Starving Time."

In autumn 1609, Captain John Smith left 500 settlers in Jamestown to return to England for treatment of a gunpowder wound. Without his stern but effective leadership, food became scarce and starvation common. According to one survivor, by spring "there remained not above sixty . . . and these most poor and miserable Creatures, preserved for the most part, by Roots, Herbs, Acorns, Walnuts, Berries, and now and then a little Fish."[6]

Lack of fresh drinking water was still another hardship. At high tide, Jamestown's water was "verie Salt," and at low tide "full of slime and filth." Their shallow well, "fed by a brackish River owzing into it," and polluted by colonists urinating or defecating too close to it, became, as one Jamestown resident observed, "the chief cause of many diseases and sicknesses which have happened to our people, who are indeed strangely afflicted with Fluxes [diarrhea]."[7]

The winter of 1609 brought severe chest infections and exposure to the cold. Summer brought malaria and dysentery.

The Pilgrims who came in December 1620, did not fare any better. Ill-prepared for the harsh New England winter, two or three settlers died each day. Within a few months, only half of their original band was still alive.[8]

Despite such wretched conditions, hundreds of settlers continued arriving, yet with no better odds of survival. By 1624, nearly 80 percent of the earliest settlers had died of starvation or disease.[9] And the average life span of those who survived was only forty years.[10]

Health among the early colonists was clearly deplorable. But for the strong, remarkably healthy Native Americans, who lacked immunity to most diseases, fate was even worse.

In 1667, for example, a sailor with smallpox landed at Accomack, Virginia. Although he was isolated by the ship's surgeons, he escaped and fled to a nearby town, where he infected two Native American groups. From there, smallpox spread all over the eastern shore with a gruesome mortality.[11]

When European colonization began, there were about one to two million Native Americans in North America.[12] Tragically, by the end of the seventeenth century, 90 percent of the Indian population had been destroyed, mostly by diseases brought over here during that period of settlement.[13]

Meanwhile, for West Africans who were forcibly enslaved, life was as harsh—and death as familiar.[14] Lying side-by-side on ships where they were mercilessly squeezed together and chained to planks and fed

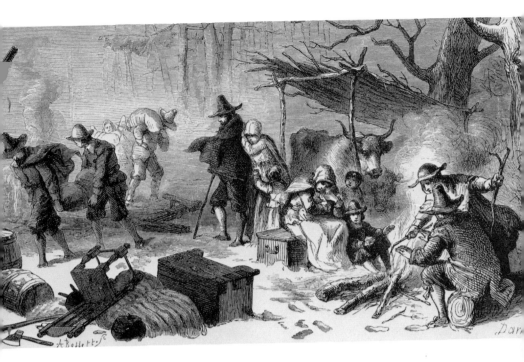

Normally, a third to half of all passengers died before they reached America. The *Mayflower*, which brought over the first Pilgrims, had only one death on board. Good fortune soon ran dry, however, because only half the Pilgrims survived their first New England winter.

hardly any food or water, as many as one-third of these West Africans died on the voyage over.[15] Then, during their brutal three-month training period in the West Indies before being shipped to the American mainland, another one-third died.[16] And the health of those who survived was seriously impaired.

Blacks had some immunity to smallpox, malaria, and yellow fever.[17] Still, they succumbed to a host of diseases brought with them from Africa, such as yaws,

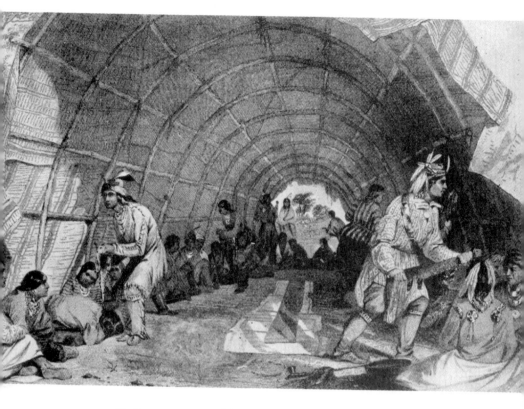

Before contact with European settlers, Native Americans had remarkably good health and strong bodies. But lacking immunity to the new germs brought here by those settlers, especially smallpox and measles, by the end of the colonial era, nearly 90 percent of them had died.

dengue, hookworm, and malaria. Indeed, life here was so wretched that poor health and death prevailed. Unaccustomed to cold winters, blacks frequently suffered severe chest colds and respiratory infections.[18] Laboring as much as twenty-one hours a day, seven days a

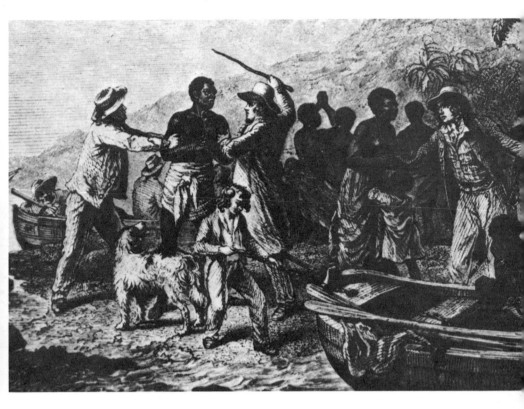

After a grueling voyage from Africa, in
deplorable conditions, slaves faced cruelty and
disgustingly inhumane treatment in America.

week, many slaves died within two or three years of
their arrival.[19]

Throughout the period, commercial ships continued bringing immigrants along with fresh supplies,
including medicine. These ships, however, also brought
disease. For example, open water buckets contained
mosquito larvae that carried malaria and yellow fever.
On unclean bodies, lice thrived and later infected set-

tlers with typhus and plague. These immigrants also spread tuberculosis, whooping cough, and influenza and helped to cause epidemics of dysentery, measles, scarlet fever, and the dreaded smallpox.

Gradually, the situation improved. Instead of four out of five newcomers dying, by 1671, four out of five were surviving.[20] Homes had been built, and land had been cleared and planted. Livestock, chickens, hens, and hogs were raised. From Native Americans, settlers had learned how to hunt and fish, and how to prepare and eat native foods such as raccoon, trout, pumpkin, corn, and maple syrup.

Repeated attacks of malaria, or "fever and *ague*," names for malaria's alternating fevers and chills, conferred some protection against the disease. And after a "seasoning" bout of the "delirious fever" that affected nearly all newcomers, the settlers developed a lifetime immunity to typhoid, the disease they got from their contaminated water supplies. Furthermore, due to an average birthrate of seven births per married woman[21] and a large pool of immigrants— Virginia alone had 100,000[22]—by 1700, the population in North America had reached 260,000 people[23] and was rapidly growing.

Unfortunately, medicine remained crude and inadequate. Poor sanitation, disease, deficient diets, and accidents continued to take their toll. Therefore, despite rapid population growth, for most colonists, old age remained a wistful goal, and sickness and death a constant companion.

## CHAPTER THREE

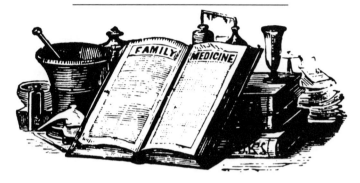

# What Ailed Them

Throughout the colonial era, maintaining health, or just trying to stay alive, was a challenge, especially during epidemics. Observing the widespread disease and death in New York City in March 1729, James Alexander wrote: "Theres no day but what theres numbers of buryings, Some of the measles but most of the pain of the Side there's hardly a house in but what had several Sick of one of the other of these Distempers."[1]

Colonial medicine was unable to cure most ailments. At times, it even worsened the patient's condition. When two-year-old Charles Drinker had a sore throat that was probably due to diphtheria, his doctor prescribed a treatment considered gentle enough. He gave Charles medicine that was only supposed to induce vomiting. Unfortunately, as the boy's mother reported in her diary, it "agatated him much and failed to work. . . . In little more than 20 minits from ye time he took it, he expired."[2]

Because colonists did not carefully record each death or know the cause of most diseases, it is impossible to give accurate and precise descriptions of what ailed them. Nearly every disease that caused a fever was diagnosed as "distemper," whereas anyone with diarrhea or abdominal cramps was diagnosed with the "flux," regardless of the cause. Likewise, the colonists would confuse one disease with another, such as syphilis with smallpox, or malaria with typhoid.

Despite these shortcomings, historians can still paint a picture of colonial disease. It is a grim one. Epidemics left a fearful mark, hitting the populace swiftly, violently, and in great numbers. A single epidemic could debilitate an entire population, and bring commerce, politics, and ordinary affairs to a virtual halt.

During New York City's 1729 measles epidemic, the New York Supreme Court was compelled to adjourn for six weeks "because of the Sickness of the town."[3] When smallpox hit only three years later, one resident reported how little business was transacted: "The Markets begin to grow very thin; the Small-Pox raging very violently in Town, which in a great measure hinders the Country People from supplying this place with Provisions."[4] When it struck southern Pennsylvania, one observer wrote: "The Living are scarce able to bury the Dead, whole Families being down at once, and many die unknown to their Neighbors."[5]

Worst of all, though, was how an epidemic ravaged the population, leaving a wake of death in its trail. Within months and even weeks, as many as 10 percent of a city's population could die.[6] With its characteristic high fever and black vomit of partially digested blood, yellow fever, or "calenture" as it was called, caused a gruesome death. One Boston resident, describing the dreaded disease, wrote: "It was a Distemper which in less than a Week's time usually carried off my neighbors with very direful Symptoms of turning *Yellow*, vomiting & bleeding every way and so Dying."[7] Small-

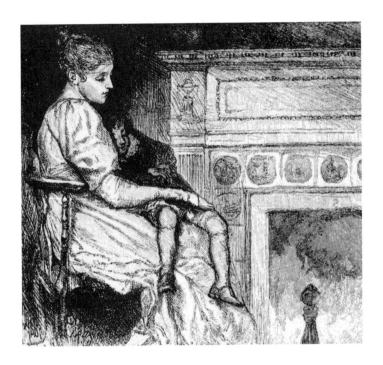

A mother comforts her child. Diseases
that are now preventable, such as measles,
smallpox, and diphtheria, killed many children
during colonial days. Some epidemics could kill
all the children in a family within weeks.

pox killed fewer of its victims than yellow fever, but
since it left so many of its survivors scarred for life, it
was feared just as much.

Among the Native Americans, who had never been
exposed to such diseases, and who therefore lacked
immunity to most of them, mortality during an epidemic was even higher. Frequently half, and occasionally all, of a group died.[8] Like many other tribes,
within two generations, the Cherokee population was

literally reduced by half. By 1780, only one-fourth of their original numbers was left.[9]

Because of their isolation, rural folk had a distinct health advantage—they were distanced from many epidemics.[10] In contrast, city dwellers, who were constantly exposed to immigrants, enslaved persons, and sailors, and faced overcrowded, unsanitary living conditions, were less fortunate. In 1793, Philadelphia lost 4,000 of its 40,000 citizens to yellow fever. When another yellow fever epidemic struck the city again only four years later, one hundred people fell ill each day, and fifty died. By the end of the epidemic, one thousand people lay buried, including nine physicians.[11]

Despite the fear epidemics aroused and the path of death they carved, they were not responsible for the majority of colonial deaths. Rather, it was endemic disease—or disease that is always around—that exacted the greatest toll on health and life in the long run. According to medical historian John Duffy, dysentery, malaria, and respiratory diseases ultimately claimed more lives than the epidemics. For even when they weren't directly responsible for death, these diseases so weakened their victims' health that they left them prone to other diseases to which they succumbed.

Dysentery, acquired mainly through spoiled food and tainted water, gave its victims painful cramps and diarrhea, and was a frequent ailment.

With its alternating high fever and chills, malaria spared few throughout the colonial period. After several bouts of malaria, however, colonists increased their resistance to it. Moreover, by the eighteenth century, malaria was limited largely to the South.

Respiratory ailments such as pleurisy, pneumonia, and influenza kept thousands of people coughing and weak, especially during the winter months, and killed thousands more.

Tuberculosis of the lungs, commonly known as "the

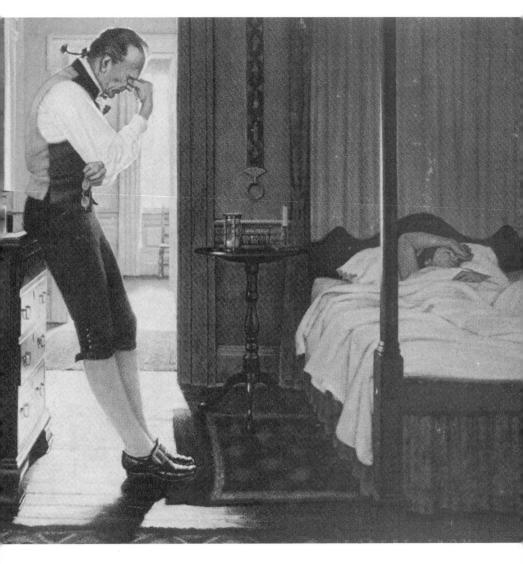

Although they lived in greater material comfort, the wealthy who lived in harbor cities, where shiploads constantly brought in foreign germs and disease, succumbed to epidemic diseases as often as their poorer brethren.

decline" or "consumption" for the way it slowly "consumes" tissue, struck numerous people. Like so many other young adults, William Drinker, the brother of Charles, became infected with tuberculosis when he was in his twenties. For years he coughed up blood-tinged phlegm and complained of soreness in his chest. Although there were times when he grew stronger, Drinker suffered from tuberculosis for over thirty years, until his death at age fifty-four.[12]

Other common diseases of the period included scarlet fever, measles, typhus, typhoid, rheumatism, dengue, diabetes, cancer, gout, and no doubt many others that colonists were unable to identify or diagnose, such as high blood pressure, appendicitis, and kidney disease.

Disease, of course, was not the only health problem. Poor obstetrics caused many women to die during childbirth, and frequent childbearing seriously impaired the health of many.[13] Martha Ballard, a skilled midwife from Maine who delivered babies in the latter part of the colonial era, earned an excellent reputation for herself. Yet nearly 1 in 200 women whom Ballard helped at childbirth died (compared to 1 in 10,000 women who die today).[14]

In addition to disease and childbirth, accidents destroyed health and claimed lives. Wooden homes often caught fire, burning their inhabitants. A fall from a horse could break a bone into a compound fracture that in colonial times required amputation. Considering that 50 percent of all amputees died of postoperative infection,[15] such accidents were clearly life threatening, and at least a serious health hazard.

Aside from Native Americans and immigrant slaves, no group had a higher mortality than infants and children. One in three children died before their second birthday,[16] and only half reached their tenth birthday.[17] Fed meager diets, spoiled food, and unpasteurized milk, they frequently suffered from dysentery and malnutrition. Lacking immunity to most germs, children fell victim to measles, diphtheria, scarlet fever, mumps, and many other diseases.

During a measles epidemic in Charleston in 1772, nine hundred children—nearly every child in the city—died.[18] As soon as an epidemic of "putrid throat distemper," or diphtheria, began in New England in 1735, mothers and fathers were "compelled to watch their children slowly strangle to death."[19] Many parents lost three, four, or five of their children at the same time. When the epidemic struck Haverhill, Massachusetts, half the town's children died and twenty-three families were left childless.[20]

Even when disease didn't kill or accidents didn't maim, poor health made its ugly mark on colonial life. In many cases, the mark was literal. "The first thing that struck every visitor to early America," observed John Josslyn, "was the bad teeth of the people. The women are pitifully tooth-shaken."[21]

In 1789, the average colonist could expect to live merely thirty-five years.[22] This number is misleading, however, because it takes into account all the infants and children who died. Actually, in the South, those who survived to their twentieth birthday could expect to live another twenty to twenty-five years. In the North, where the climate was healthier and there was less disease, twenty year olds could expect to live another thirty or so years.[23]

Furthermore, considering their widespread disease and ill health, many Americans lived incredibly long lives compared to Europeans. Registers in Woodstock, Connecticut, in the 1780s show that more than 1 out of 9 residents was an octogenarian or older. Yet a comparable community in France that same year had only 1 in 42 residents who reached such longevity.[24]

Another way to understand the American advantage is to look at the yearly death rate. In 1781, Salem, Massachusetts, was one of the most unhealthy towns in New England. Still, only 1 in 50 Salem residents died that year, compared to 1 in 30 who died in Paris, 1 in 23 who died in London, and 1 in 24 who died in rural France.[25] "From all the facts," wrote eighteenth-century French journalist Brissot de Warville, "it must be concluded that life is much longer in the United States of America, than in the most salubrious countries of Europe."[26]

Based on a report of vital statistics, de Warville determined that "America was not a place of excessive disease, nor short life expectancy. Contrary, it was a place of rapid increase and long life."[27]

Such observations are, of course, relative to the times. By today's standards, disease was excessive and life was short. It is only natural to question why this was so.

Until the discovery of germs, effective treatment, or preventive medicine, most of what ailed colonists was untreatable or unavoidable. One of the colonists' biggest problems, though, was ignorance.

Ignorant of medicine, they failed to cure most ailments, and frequently inflicted harm on themselves when they tried. Unaware of germs they could not see, they spread infection. Unaware of the causes of diseases, they spread diseases themselves.

In 1735, Susannah Wilson had diphtheria. Aware of her impending death, Wilson gave her possessions to her older sisters. Then she "took her children in her arms and kiss'd them."[28] But her kiss was probably the kiss of death. For unbeknownst to Wilson, diphtheria is highly contagious and spread through direct contact.

Ignorant of personal hygiene, colonists rarely washed. Their dirty bodies, clothing, and bedsheets

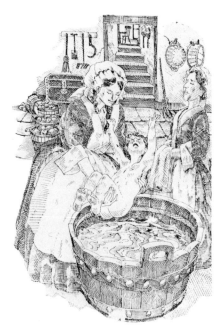

*Left:* Given the colonists' misconception that bathing is bad because it might open the pores to disease, colonists rarely bathed. Few probably felt deprived, though, since bathing meant a plunge into icy cold water pumped from the well.

*Below:* Unlike the English and French colonists, Native Americans had a healthy view of bathing. Birthing huts like this were often set up near running streams or by the seashore, so women could bathe after giving birth.

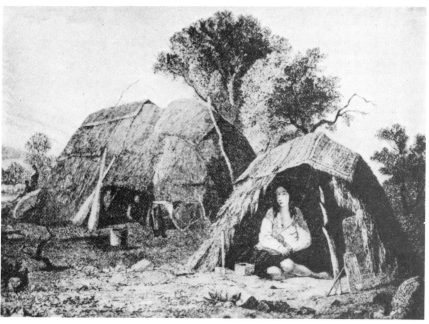

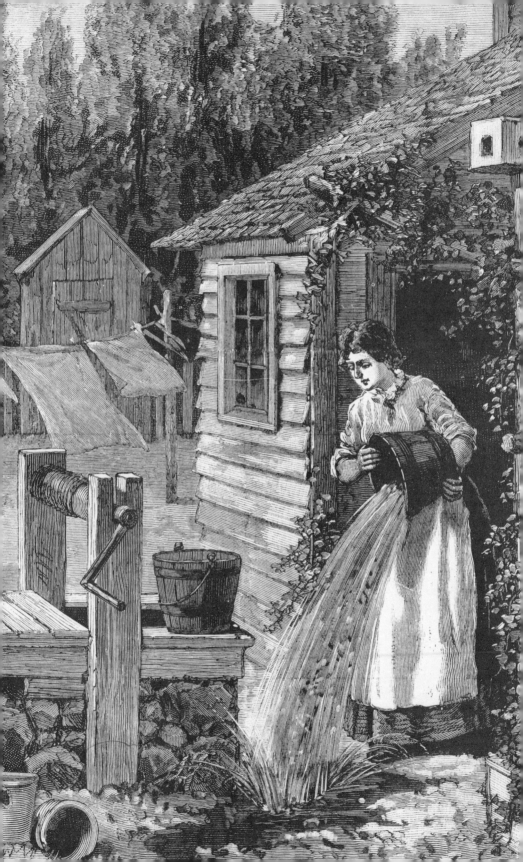

harbored vermin and bacteria that infected them with disease.

Ignorant of sanitation, colonists let dead carcasses rot in their streets, garbage pollute their harbors, and human waste taint their wells. Few cities had sewage systems or garbage collection.

Ignorant of nutrition, colonists ate too much, and much of what they ate was unbalanced, sometimes spoiled, and too salty. To wash down their food, they drank copious quantities of hard cider, ale, and other alcoholic beverages.

Clearly, colonial health faced a formidable challenge from a number of foes: widespread disease, poor nutrition, little sanitation, accidents, war, and difficult childbirths. During an epidemic, rich and poor, male and female alike fell victim. Overall, while some groups fared better than others, none could take good health for granted.

Ignorance played a huge role in colonial disease. This woman is throwing her dirty household water near the family well, where it will seep underground and contaminate the drinking water. Nor does she know to boil the water to make it safe for drinking.

## CHAPTER FOUR

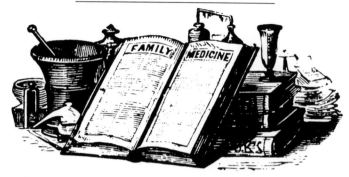

# What They Knew
# and What They Didn't Know

John Todd was a medical student during colonial times. He had never dissected a body. "Oh if I could have had a skeleton to look at for a single hour," he lamented in his memoirs.

Soon that desire came true. Wasting no time after he overheard a hunter mention a recently buried corpse in the nearby woods, Todd hastily rushed off to find it. Within three days, he had unburied the cadaver, taken it apart, and closely examined it. "Three days hard work and work not the most pleasant," he later remarked.

"I gloated over those bones! studied them! strung them! They were the beginning of my professional knowledge."[1] They were also illegally obtained. Body snatching and dissecting human cadavers were strictly taboo and against the law. As late as 1820, in fact, the people in one New Hampshire village voted never to sponsor a physician who had ever participated in human dissection or autopsy.[2]

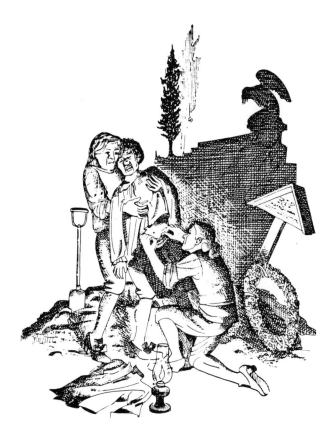

Because a taboo kept doctors from legally
obtaining dead bodies to dissect, many
used cadavers stolen from graves.

At times, public opinion toward dissection even
grew hostile. A few young surgeons at New York Hospital rather defiantly dangled a partially dissected limb
from a window, calling to a young boy below that the
limb belonged to his recently deceased mother. When
the boy's father learned of the incident, he was so out-
raged that he gathered together a mob that rioted for
four days against the medical establishment.[3]

Doctors occasionally viewed a portion of the body through an open wound. Yet until they studied anatomy by dissecting dead bodies, how the body worked remained a mystery. Given such mystery, there was little fact to colonial medicine, and much fiction. Nonetheless, theories based on fiction became the bulwark of colonial medical thought.

During the Renaissance in Europe—a period from the 1300s to the 1600s—art, literature, and learning soared. Interest in ancient Greek doctors was part of this mental expansion. Students of "physick," as medicine was called, enthusiastically studied medical texts that had been translated into Latin, the language of European scholars.

The most widely read Greek medical authors were Hippocrates and Galen, neither of whom had ever dissected a human body. By working on animals, Galen had learned something about anatomy (our body's structure) and physiology (the way the body works). But without human dissection, Galen still knew very little. His ignorance, however, did not keep him from believing that he knew a great deal. In fact, Galen wrote over three hundred medical treatises, including a book on anatomy that became popular among Renaissance scholars.

Based on the Greek philosopher Aristotle's belief that everything in the physical world is made up of only four basic substances, Galen concluded that the human body has four basic elements, or "*humors,*" as he named them. He determined that the body's secretions, which he named phlegm, blood, yellow bile, and black bile, were these four basic humors. How wrong he was. Modern chemistry teaches us that there are 106 elements, not merely 4.

Since Galen had never dissected a sinus cavity where phlegm (mucous) is actually produced, he mistakenly claimed that phlegm comes from the brain.

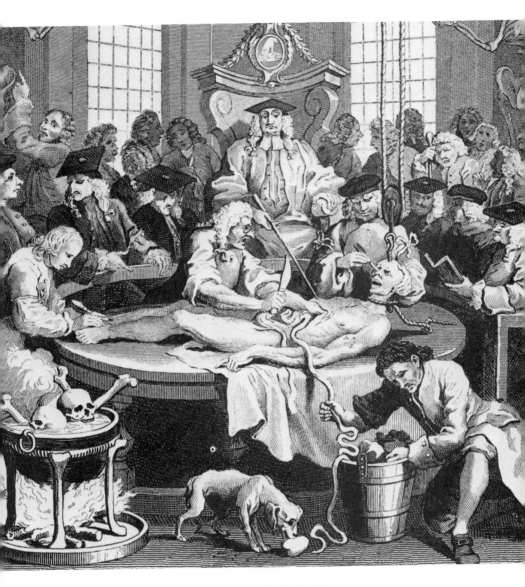

In this woodcut, titled *The Reward of Cruelty,* artist William Hogarth pokes fun at the medical professor trying to teach his class anatomy.

Likewise, he erroneously believed that blood, which the body produces in our bone marrow, is from the heart, and that yellow and black bile come from the liver and spleen, respectively.

According to Galen's theory of humors, good health required that the "four elements" be in perfect balance, a balance he also believed changes with each season. Furthermore, he thought that anything disturbing the balance, from weather changes to overeating, caused disease to set in.

To treat disease, Galen advised methods he believed could restore balance to the humors. For example, an "excess" of blood, which he believed was indicated by a strong pulse and a fever, needed to be reduced by bleeding the patient of the excess. Similarly, an "excess" of bile required purging through emetics or vomiting.

As early as the sixteenth century, a few doctors began to criticize Galen's theories. Swiss alchemist Paracelsus argued that there was no basis to humors, that instead, our basic elements are chemicals. Strong criticism also came from a bold Flemish physician, Andreas Vesalius, who defied the Church's taboo against dissection and dared to look inside the human body.

With only his naked eye, Vesalius studied human anatomy by using probes and other crude instruments and encouraged his medical students to follow suit. When his elegantly illustrated book, *De Humani Corporis Fabrica Libri Septem*, was published in Europe in 1543 to acclaim and acceptance, medical science began to climb out of its Dark Ages.

During the colonial period, other doctors and scholars blazed the way to further anatomical discoveries. The English physician William Harvey discovered the circulation of blood. Anton van Leeuwenhoek, a Dutch linen draper who had an interest in medicine, constructed a simple microscope, and for the first time in history viewed single-celled organisms such as red corpuscles and spermatozoa. Marcello Malpighi, an Italian anatomist, peered through such a microscope to discover red capillaries.

Yet, despite these medical discoveries, and the sharp criticism of Parcelsus, Vesalius, and others, until the nineteenth century, Galenic theory reigned supreme.

Although Galen made some remarkable discoveries, such as the diaphragm's role in breathing, his reputation rested on his humoral theory of medicine. More than fifteen centuries after Galen died, humoral theory remained medical gospel. And why not? With a continuing taboo against dissection, few medical scholars knew enough to prove Galen wrong.

Given how incorrect colonial doctors were about anatomy, they scored rather poorly on their knowledge of disease. Using his microscope, Leeuwenhoek had identified single-celled organisms that he named "animalcules." But two more centuries passed before anyone realized that many of these minute organisms were germs that caused certain diseases. Nor were colonists aware of other causes of disease, such as inadequate diets, viruses, or glandular disorders.

Sometimes their speculation about disease came close to the truth, but rarely close enough. For example, the colonists believed that marshes and swamps emitted a bad vapor, or "miasma," that infects people with diseases such as yellow fever and malaria,[4] when mosquitoes are actually to blame.

After Isaac Newton discovered a universal law of physics, medical scholars sought a universal theory that would explain disease. Herman Boerhaave, for example, maintained that every disease came from an imbalance of "natural activities."[5] London physician John Brown concluded that all disease comes from an imbalance of tension in the blood—either too much blood, which he called *sthenic*, or too little, which he termed *asthenic*. Like his Galenic colleagues, Brown advocated bleeding, purging, vomiting, sweating, or blistering to correct the imbalance.

Benjamin Rush was sure he had found the most simple, concise system of medicine the world had yet seen. "Be not startled, Gentlemen," he said in a speech, "follow me and I will say that there is but one disease in the world,"[6] which he concluded was too much tension or pressure in the veins. For his "one disease," he had one basic remedy—copious bleeding.

Deeply religious people like the Puritans blamed disease on the Almighty, suggesting that it was God's punishment for sins and wrongdoings. Similarly, Native Americans and African Americans viewed sickness as the result of transgressions against the gods, or God.[7]

Some people even blamed disease on the constellations, voodoo, and other superstitions. One of the most popular and beloved doctors of his time, Englishman Nicholas Culpeper used astrology as the basis for his medical practice and advice.

Defying the quest for a single cause of disease, seventeenth-century English physician Thomas Sydenham searched for many causes. Disease, he suggested, could be classified much the way botanists had classified the plant world. Furthermore, once a specific disease was pinpointed, Sydenham was sure that its remedy could be found. He blamed disease on particles in the air "that enter the body and taint the blood," and on "decay of the humors."[8]

As we have already learned, building medical theory based on Galen's four humors had little chance of reaching medical truth. In 1771, after performing hundreds of autopsies, Italian physician Giovanni Morgagni attributed disease to specific organs or structures within the body. Writing that "symptoms are the cry of the suffering organ," Morgagni insisted that it was useless to seek the cause of disease among the humors.9

Sydenham and Morgagni successfully identified a few specific diseases. Yet most afflictions remained unclassified, largely because they were so difficult to diagnose at the time. For with no knowledge of germs or viruses or of how organs malfunction, and without being able to test the blood or spinal fluid or scan the bone and tissues, how could colonists improve their guesswork? The fact was that most colonial practitioners, lacking even the basic diagnostic tools, could not.

Although there was never a shortage of theories about disease during the colonial period, there was a lack of medical truth. Ill health and disease were attributed to many causes—from the weather and bad vapors in the air to overeating and wrongful behavior. Rarely did healers pinpoint the real villains, and because they didn't, disease spread.

Unaware of germs, colonial practitioners knew nothing about antiseptics or hygiene. With contaminated hands and unsterile instruments, they pulled teeth, sawed off limbs, and internally examined pregnant women, spreading their germs and infecting their patients—often fatally.

Eventually, medical scholarship began eroding Galen's influence, and new theories replaced the old ones. Unfortunately, most of these new theories were as full of holes as the old ones.

## CHAPTER FIVE

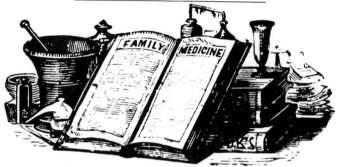

# A Sorry State of Affairs

**Y**ou're living in colonial America, and you have a terrible toothache. Your head throbs with pain. For several days you have put "a little piece of opium as big as a great pinnes head into the hollow place of the Akeing tooth."[1]

Contrary to the doctor's claim that this treatment never fails, it does. Your tooth still aches, and you are desperate to try something else.

You can have the tooth drilled. But in colonial days, this will be painful, expensive, and more time consuming than having your tooth pulled. Therefore, like most colonists, you opt to treat the toothache by getting rid of the tooth causing it.

With his knife, the tooth puller cuts around your gum. Then, using a turnkey device, he grabs your aching tooth and tries to yank it out. It doesn't quite work. To gain more leverage, he presses his knee on your chest, then gives a twist and another strong pull. Job's done.

Although it was painful, and occasionally caused infection, pulling teeth was effective—it cured the toothache, after all. Other medical treatments were far less effective, and sometimes worse, than the ailments they were supposed to cure.

In order to diagnose an illness, the famous Dr. Sydenham advised carefully observing a patient's symptoms. But without clinical thermometers, fevers could not be accurately diagnosed. Without X-ray machines, seeing most broken bones, tumors, and other internal problems was impossible. Without watches with second hands, pulses went unmeasured. Without knowledge of percussion—tapping the chest to detect problems like pneumonia or asthma—doctors had trouble diagnosing respiratory ailments. And without stethoscopes, heart murmurs and irregularities went undetected.

Added to their lack of diagnostic tools came the colonial practitioners' ignorance of the real causes of diseases. Thus, even if they could accurately diagnose symptoms, without knowing their cause, treatment resembled a game of roulette.

Despite their shortcomings, colonial healers had a storehouse of medical treatments. Some practitioners even believed that they could find a cure for any medical disorder.[2] They also believed that the treatment ought to match the disease. "Desperate diseases require desperate remedies," wrote Dr. Benjamin Rush of Philadelphia when he resolved to "take whatever measures are necessary to save a patient's life."[3]

To treat the high fever and bloody vomiting characteristic of Philadelphia's yellow fever epidemic in 1793, Dr. Rush recommended powerful calomel purges and bleeding patients of more than six or eight pints of blood over a two-or three-day period—nearly ten times the safety limit for healthy blood donors.[4]

Not all healers were as compulsive as Dr. Rush in their treatment. A few prescribed more moderate treatments, choosing to rely on the healing power of nature. As Dr. Rush was purging and bleeding his yellow fever

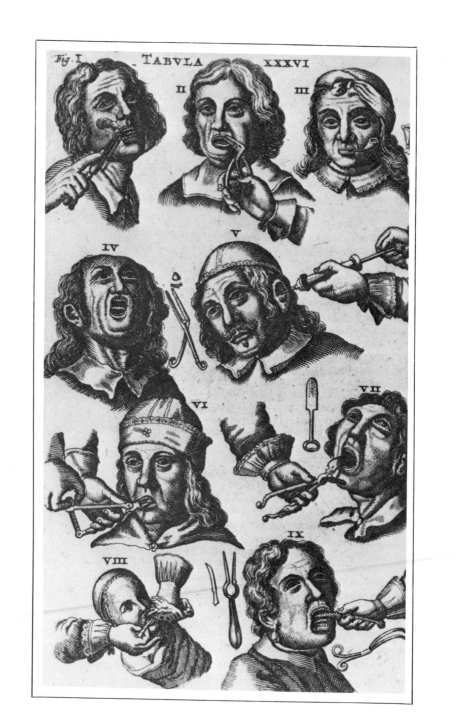

patients, Dr. Adam Kuhn, a colleague of Dr. Rush's in Philadelphia, recommended a gentle course of bark (quinine), camomile tea, cold baths, and wine.[5] Likewise, Dr. James Currie advocated personal hygiene, plenty of fresh air, and making patients as comfortable as possible[6]—sound advice, even today.

For the most part, though, because of their misconceptions of how the body worked, treatments were usually ineffective, inappropriate, and sometimes dangerous. Rather than prescribe a cool bath to lower a fever, for example, doctors advised their patients to stay under layers of blankets until they sweated the fever out. Unaware that tuberculosis requires rest, doctors told patients to ride horseback as much as possible. Ignorant that germs cause sore throats and common colds, doctors blistered patients on the neck and back (to force out the "bad vapor"). And believing that blood is replenished in hours, not weeks, these doctors drew too much.

Most treatment sought to correct the "imbalance of humors" by ridding the body of its "excess fluids." Doctors interpreted fevers and strong pulses as evidence of an excess of blood, a condition that they concluded required bleeding. Likewise, they believed that any vomiting required treatment to induce even more vomiting in order to balance the bile. In July 1788, seventeen-year-old Sally Drinker had dysentery.

This engraving shows various methods of curing a toothache. Although patients probably took a drug to lessen the pain, without anesthetics, a visit to the dentist no doubt caused much anxiety.

Though she was "very ill with vomiting and flux . . ." and had "above 30 stools a day," she was given an enema, three spoonfuls of castor oil, and a dose of rhubarb.[7]

Commenting on the heroic treatments of his day (for many treatments were rather rigorous or "heroic," for it often took a hero to withstand them), Dr. William Douglass of Boston remarked, "It was very uniform— bleeding, vomiting, blistering, purging, anodyne, et cetera. If the illness continued, there was repetendi, and finally murderandi."[8]

That Dr. Rush had embraced bleeding as the choice treatment is no surprise. Throughout colonial times, and far into the nineteenth century, bleeding patients was very common.

First, a lancet (small knife) was used to cut open a vein, or a scarificator (metal box encasing a group of small spring-loaded blades) was used to put several cuts in the skin. Next, a heated cup was placed on the cut vein or skin. As the cup cooled, a vacuum formed that caused the blood to flow more freely. Often blood was drawn until the patient became faint, or even unconscious.

Sometimes the heated cup was used without cutting a vein. It drew blood under the skin's surface and was called "dry cupping."

Another popular method of drawing blood was leeching. Parasitic invertebrates, or leeches, which are found in rivers and streams, were used for areas that were difficult to bleed with cups, like the eyes, mouth, and anus.

After the patient's skin was washed and shaved, a drop of milk or blood was used to encourage the leech to suck. Once enough blood was drawn—each leech was capable of one ounce (which took an hour)—it was removed by sprinkling it with salt or a solution of vinegar (which also caused the leech to regurgitate so it could be used again sooner).

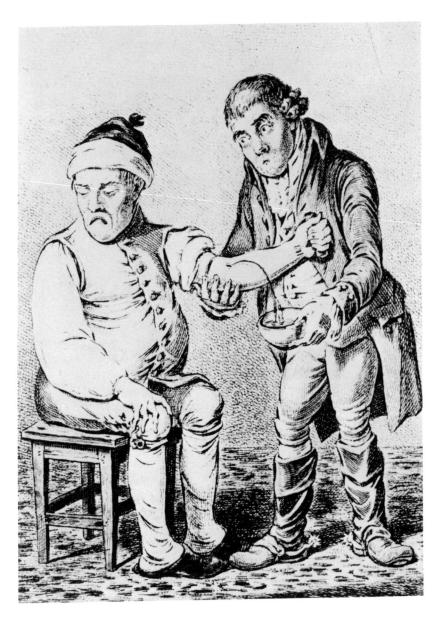

Colonial doctors had a penchant for bloodletting,
regarding it as proper treatment for just about
any ailment, from nervous tension to yellow fever.

Leeches were stored in jars at doctors' offices or at the shops of blacksmiths, barbers, and apothecaries—wherever bloodletting was done.

The primary reason for phlebotomy's popularity is that in the short run, at least, it worked; it could reduce a fever and lower high blood pressure. The danger, though, was an excessive blood loss, a drop in blood pressure, or infection resulting from unsterile instruments.

A common theory during the colonial era was that the body could only contain one illness at a time. If a second illness entered, the first would leave. This theory inspired another popular treatment—blistering—which was often used along with bloodletting, particularly for colds and other respiratory infections. To blister the skin, doctors applied hot pokers or a plaster of ground cantharides, or dried beetles, that burned the skin and forced it to blister.

Another frequently used heroic treatment was inducing the patient to purge his or her bowels or to vomit (emesis). The most popular cathartics used to empty the bowels and emetics used to induce vomiting included calomel, tartar, and saltpeter.

During the seventeenth century, a theory that the primary cause of human disease is constipation inspired still another treatment—clysters. Using a large and formidable syringe, called a clyster (enema), colonists emptied their bowels.

The danger of purging and vomiting, of course, was that it caused many patients to become dangerously dehydrated and weak. Drugs like calomel, though they were somewhat effective, caused sore gums, tooth loss, and acute (serious) mercury poisoning.

Colonists also believed in the medicinal power of "sweating out an illness." Patients with fevers were bundled under layers of blankets until their fever broke with a sweat. Camphor and saltpeter (potassium nitrate) were considered effective for "calming fevers and delirium."9

Although the practice was never too popular among European settlers, Native Americans "drove out the evil spirits" in sweat lodges that were much like our modern saunas. In the center of a tightly closed-off tent or tepee, the healer drenched hot stones with water, causing a thick steam to form. When patients were covered with sweat, they plunged into cold water. Afterward, their bodies were massaged. Then they took a long nap.

In addition to treatments that "balanced the humors" or eliminated the "bad vapors," colonial doctors relied on surgery mostly to treat wounds, broken and dislocated bones, and skin abscesses and ulcers. Sometimes doctors trepanned the skull, which involved cutting out a piece of it to relieve pressure from the brain. However, most healers avoided major surgery on the head, chest, and abdomen.10 For without sterile operating conditions and antiseptics to prevent infection, without effective painkillers, and without effective ways to control excessive bleeding, surgery was painful, dangerous, and often fatal.

To deal with their pain during surgery, patients took large doses of opium or rum. When drugs or liquor were unavailable, patients might be given a bullet or stick to bite down on. Or they were given nothing. Of course, there was still so much pain to endure that patients had to be physically restrained. A great number of frightened patients went into shock and died. Many others survived the ordeal, only to die shortly afterward from infections caused by unsterile instruments and dressings.

Along with the traditional treatment methods, treatment fads came and went. One of the most distinguished eighteenth-century quacks, Dr. Elisha Perkins, talked hundreds of people into using his metallic forks to cure their ills. "These consisted of two instruments, one having the appearance of steel, the other of brass," wrote one of his critics, "and the mysterious influence with which Elisha and his son claimed they could permeate the true Perkinean Tractors was in reality an endowment from the minds of willing patients."[11]

In the eighteenth century, when Italian physician Luigi Galvani discovered that muscle tissue responded to electricity, a keen interest in static electrical treatment arose. Static electricity was used to treat a range of disorders, including blindness, cancer, consumption, dropsy, dysentery, gallstones, palsy, syphilis, and worms.[12] By the late 1700s, physicians were using electricity at the Public Hospital in Williamsburg, Virginia, to treat mental illness.

As the range of treatment options indicates, colonists did not lack ways of *doing* something about their medical problems. Alas, treatments such as bleeding, blistering, vomiting, purging, and ingesting excessive amounts of ineffective or dangerous remedies kept colonial medicine in a sorry state of affairs.

# CHAPTER SIX

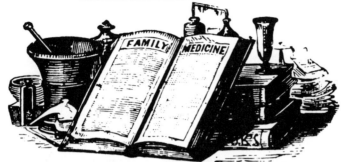

# And the Medicine Goes Down

For a chill, Dr. Zorobbabel Endicot of Salem, Massachusetts, recommended taking "the Drye shell of a Turtell, and beat smale & boyled in water. While 2 thirds of the water be consumed, drinke of it 2 or 3 times."[1] Although it may sound less appetizing than a bowl of homemade chicken soup, preparing turtle broth was simple enough, and drinking the hot broth during a chill was probably quite soothing.

For itching, Dr. Ball of Northboro, Massachusetts, gave this recipe: one quart of fish worms, washed; one pound of hog's lard, stewed and filtered; half a pint of turpentine; and half a pint of good brandy. Mix these ingredients together, and simmer well.[2]

Recipes for such common remedies were passed down as family traditions or found in books. One of the most popular books was written by English herbalist and physician, Nicholas Culpeper. First published in 1708, his book *The English Physician*, more commonly known as *The Complete Herbal*, was so popular that it went into dozens of reprints. Early settlers consulted it widely, not only for medical advice but also to find out the most auspicious times for planting and harvesting their crops.

Apothecaries and other purveyors of medicine were sources of more than two hundred drugs,[3] which consisted of a variety of ingredients from plants and metals to dung and urine. Many drugs had to be imported and were therefore quite expensive. To substitute for the most costly ingredients, colonists turned to simpler, cheaper ones found in their households, gardens, and woods.

Colonial households contained ingredients such as vinegar, flour, and the old standby, chicken soup.[4] From colonial gardens came herbs like foxglove, sweet basil, and sassafras. Rhubarb, green beans, onions, and currants were also used.

Herbs were classified into two groups—benefits and simples. Benefits were plants used for prevention, and simples were plants used for cures. For example, rose hips, which was used to *prevent* scurvy, was classified as a benefit, whereas black walnut hulls, which were used to *cure* tapeworm, were classified as a simple. Garlic was considered both a benefit and a simple because it was used to stimulate the digestive system as well as to cure asthma, whooping cough, and heart problems.[5]

In the sixteenth century, Swiss alchemist and physician Paracelsus, who had criticized Galen's medical theories, developed the idea that every plant was "signed" by God with a clue to its medical use. According to his Doctrine of Signatures, or just "similars," as it was also called, the body part a plant is supposed to be able to cure can be determined by the plant's shape, color, or scent, or the habitat it resembles. For instance, walnut meat resembles brain tissue, so according to Paracelsus, it can cure brain disease. Likewise, flowers that look like bright eyes are considered good optical remedies, and juicy plants, such as lettuce or figs, are supposed to help nursing mothers.[6]

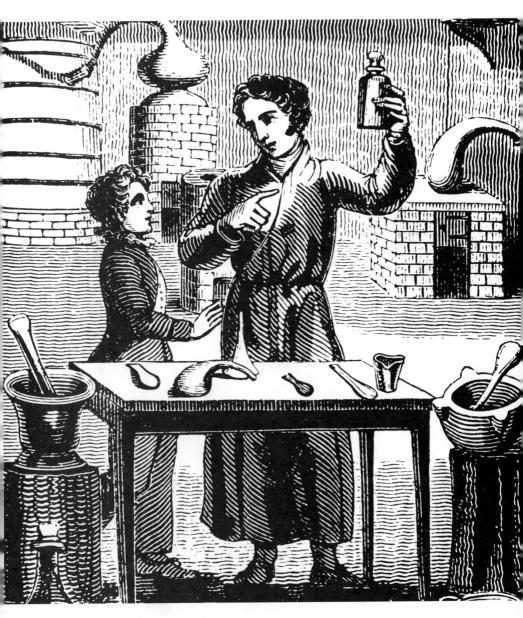

To learn a medical trade such as apothecary,
young boys apprenticed themselves to
a master for several years.

Paracelsus also introduced metals into pharmacopoeia (a group of available drugs). These included lead, sulfur, iron, arsenic, copper sulfate, and potassium sulfate.[7] As we learned in the previous chapter, mercury in the form of mercury chloride or calomel was widely used. Two other chemicals that gained popularity were Glauber's salt and Epsom salts (magnesium sulfate), which are still in use today.

Many colonists also believed that at the geographic site of an illness its treatment could be found, and they therefore searched for native remedies. Some of the earliest and most popular native "finds" were sassafras and tobacco.[8] "Tobacco helps digestions, the Gout, the Tooth-Ache, prevents infection by scents," wrote John Josselyn in 1674, as he extolled the virtues of tobacco. "It heals the cold and cools them that sweat, feedeth the hungry, spent spirits restoreth, purgeth the stomach, killith nits and lice."[9]

In addition to relying on traditional medicines, colonists discovered new ones through the empirical method. If they tried a remedy that appeared effective, they used it again and recommended it as well.

Still other medicines were made according to secret recipes and sold commercially as "patent medicines." These included brand names such as Scot's Pills, Daffy's Elixir, Dutch Drops, Goddards Drops, and Seignettes Salts, to name a few.[10] Sometimes, these patent medicines contained powerful narcotics, such as opium, which helped patients feel better, but which also became addictive.

Colonial medicine often contained repulsive ingredients, as the following diary entry by an eighteenth-century midwife reveals: "I was called Early this morn to see Lidia Savage who was very ill. . . . Gave her some urin and honeey & some Liquoris & put a plaster to her stomach. Went up afternoon. Find her Relieved."[11] Even Reverend Cotton Mather, one of Boston's leading medical authorities, advocated such ingredients. "Hu-

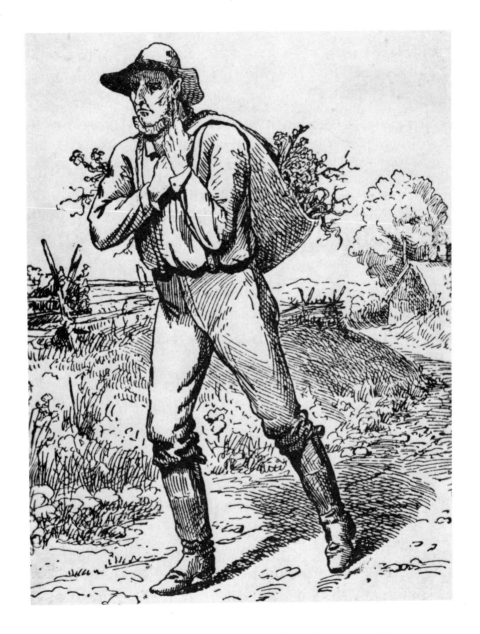

Rural doctors scouted the woods and countryside,
relying on their gardens to supply most of the
medicinal herbs, such as sassafras and digitalis.

man excreta," he enthusiastically declared, "is a remedy for Human Bodies that is hardley to be paralleled ... and urine has virtues far beyond all the water of medicinal springs."[12]

Many colonial remedies, such as snakeroot, dittany, senna, lemnian earth, alum, sweet gums, and tobacco, have no medicinal value,[13] seem preposterous, and like tobacco, are even harmful. Still, although these remedies have probably been replaced today with better drugs, a few of them were actually effective.

Colonists learned from Native Americans that they could lessen their pain by chewing the inside bark of the willow tree, which contained an ingredient that goes into our modern-day aspirin.[14]

The drug opium was used in a variety of ways, from pain relief to tranquilizer. Like calomel, opium had a dangerous side effect—namely addiction. Since opium also had few rivals, though, it was extremely popular. "Opium is an article which no physician ought ever to want," advised Dr. Thaddeus Betts in 1778. "It is so extensively useful, and in cases so perilous and urgent, where no substitute will supply its defect, that physicians ... would be lame and deficient without it."[15] Dr. Betts ensured his own supply of opium by growing and harvesting poppies, a practice he highly recommended.[16]

One of the few drug discoveries of colonial times was the bark of the cinchona tree, native to the Andes Mountains in Peru, South America. Called by various names—Peruvian bark, Jesuit's bark, countess power, or simply, "the bark"—it is highly effective against malaria.

Other effective herbs discovered by colonists included digitalis, opium poppy, and ipecac. Unfortunately, because many of these herbs worked so well for certain symptoms and diseases, they were also widely used for many that they did not help at all.[17]

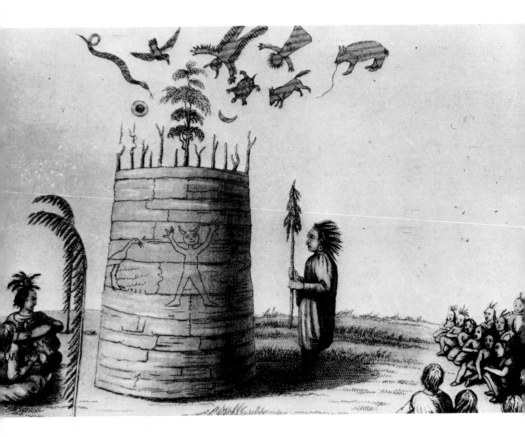

Lodge of a Midiwine prophet during initiation
ceremony. As he passed from lodge to lodge,
the initiate learned more and more of the
medicinal qualities of certain herbs.

In the end, as Andrew Duncan of Edinburgh, Scotland, has suggested, many adult patients recovered no
matter what their treatment course had been.[18] But
given the loathsome nature of so much of colonial
medicine, as well as its danger, such positive outcomes
are all the more astonishing.

## CHAPTER SEVEN

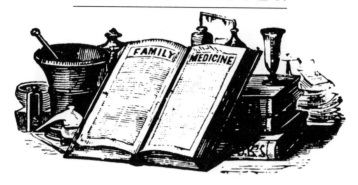

# Healers

Peter Bryant grew up with medicine since his father was a doctor. When Bryant was old enough, his father showed him how to mix powders, make pills, bleed patients, apply poultices, and do what he could to heal the sick and injured.

In 1792, Bryant gave himself the title "Doctor" and began practicing medicine in Bridgewater, Connecticut. "With my small stock of book knowledge," wrote the young Dr. Bryant of his medical background, "without experience in the ways of the world, my whole property consisting of a horse, a few books, about $25 worth of medicine, I launched out into the world to begin business."[1]

Twenty years later, Bryant was still haunted by his inadequate education. Referring to a patient whose worsening condition he was unable to correctly diagnose, Bryant lamented, "I have been wholly unable to satisfy myself as to the cause of his death."[2]

Unlike Dr. Bryant, physicians today have a college and medical school education, have passed exams testing their medical knowledge, and are members of medical associations that set professional standards. During most of the colonial era, however, the training and standards for doctors were very different.

Anyone could simply read about medicine and learn enough to become a doctor. Or a person could learn to be a doctor by apprenticing to someone who already practiced medicine. Anyone with the tools to amputate—and the guts to do so—could become a doctor. People with a knack for gardening and mixing concoctions could prepare remedies and sell them. Anyone eager to deliver babies could become a midwife. Remarkably, anyone with any interest in medicine could practice it.

"Quacks abound like locusts in Egypt," wrote William Smith in 1757, observing the widespread lack of training. "Any man at his pleasure sets up for physicians, apothecary, and surgeon. No candidates are either examined, licensed, or sworn to fair practice."[3]

As soon as the first European settlers arrived, they were accompanied by physicians or "chirurgeons" (surgeons). To "comfort the sick," the Dutch East India Company sent men who had trained at Holland's famous medical school in Leyden. Fifteen "physicians of prominence" were listed among Virginia's early settlers, including Dr. Lawrence Bohun, who served for eleven years before his death in 1621. Over thirty physicians, including Deacon Samuel Fuller, one of the original Pilgrims to settle Plymouth, served the Massachusetts Bay Colony in the first 150 years.[4]

These healers were accompanied by midwives, surgeons, and other practitioners. And, of course, Native Americans already had healers, called shamans, among their people.

For the most part, well-educated men of high social status had little reason to endure the hardships and

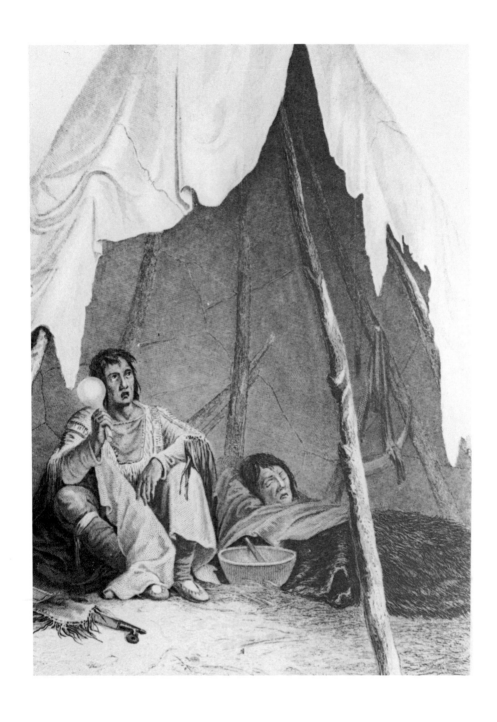

uncertainties of the colonies. Or, like Dr. Thomas Wotton, the Surgeon General to Jamestown in 1610, they returned home to Europe in a short while.

On the other hand, healers of lesser social status did come, for the same reasons thousands of others immigrated—better opportunities. Who were these healers, and where did they learn to heal?

During the seventeenth and eighteenth centuries, medicine was a subject that university students studied. Most universities were run by the Church, which maintained a taboo against touching human blood or dissecting human cadavers. Thus, even though students *learned* about medicine, they had little clinical experience with it.

When many of these university graduates entered the clergy and came to America, they found that even their spartan medical background proved useful. Some of the most progressive medical thinking of the era, in fact, can be credited to two Boston ministers—Reverends Peter Thacher and Cotton Mather.

Thacher's sensible guide to treating smallpox advised a moderate regime that included fresh air in the sick room and cooling medicine to bring down fever, both innovations for his time.[5] To Cotton Mather's credit goes the first American treatise on medical prac-

Native American shamans tried to heal both the body and the soul. This Winnebago medicine man has just administered an herbal medicine and perhaps helped his patient "sweat" out the illness. Now he is calling on the Great Spirit to heal him.

tice, *The Angel of Bethesda*, and the adoption of small-pox inoculation.

Laypersons made significant medical contributions. Ben Franklin invented bifocals, identified the cause of lead poisoning, and helped found Pennsylvania Hospital.

Although women were denied a formal education, some women took a keen interest in medicine, learning it from books and experience. Indeed, until men encroached on obstetrics in the latter part of the colonial period, women assisted at childbirth and provided most of the home care for the sick and wounded. As Laurel Thatcher Ulrich reports in her book, *A Midwife's Tale*, women like Merriam Pollard of Maine swabbed tonsils, changed dressings, applied plasters, and administered clysters (enemas). And if their patients died, they "eased their eyelids and limbs into sleeplike dignity."[6]

The most famous midwife of colonial times was Anne Hutchinson, who actually earned her reputation as a religious leader. In 1637, Hutchinson began hosting religious meetings in her Boston home, where she feverishly spoke out. When her derogatory remarks about Boston's ministers reached Massachusetts colony's Governor John Winthrop, the irate leader banished Hutchinson from the colony. With her husband and children, Hutchinson fled to the more religiously tolerant colony of Rhode Island and founded Portsmouth, near Newport.

Childbirth and dying took place largely at home. And since colonial families were huge, their members were on intimate terms with both.

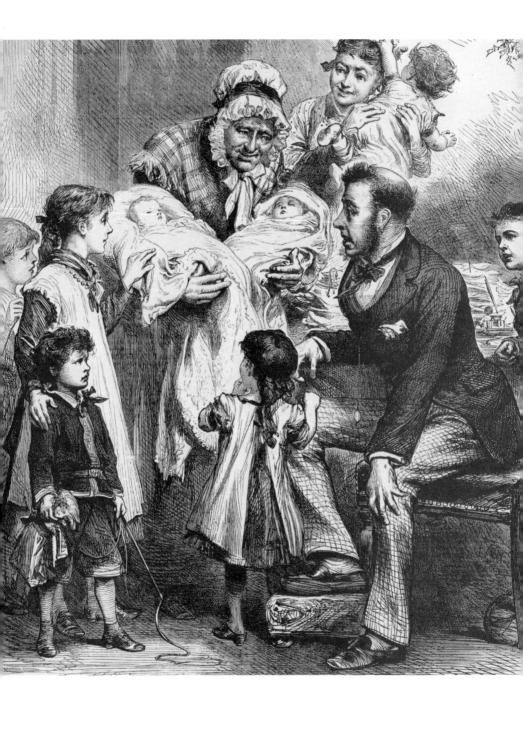

During the years that followed, scores of midwives were among those condemned as witches by colonial leaders eager to "purge their community of the devil." In 1692, at the height of colonial religious fanaticism, over one hundred people were imprisoned for witchcraft, including a number of midwives, many of whom were hung or burned at the stake.[7]

Although they were separated from European tradition, Native American healers were esteemed by those who valued their closeness to nature. According to historian William Postell, even those who *claimed* to have knowledge of Native American lore were popular.[8]

In Great Britain, physicians traditionally left the "dirty work" of amputation, tooth extraction, bloodletting, and the like to people of lesser social status. Those who took on such work were called "chirurgeons" (surgeons), and if they were barbers, they were called "barber-chirurgeons." Nor did physicians or surgeons stoop to mix or sell medicine. That became the province of apothecaries (druggists).

Trade unions, or guilds, which licensed members in each of these professions, guaranteed that the lines separating each of them remained well drawn. Because of a shortage of physicians and apothecaries, however, such distinctions were difficult to draw in America.

Out of necessity physicians amputated limbs, pulled teeth, and dispensed medicine. Apothecaries bled customers. Surgeons took on the work of physicians and called themselves Doctor. In addition to delivering babies, midwives dispensed medicine and treated the sick.

In 1765, Dr. John Morgan, one of the founders of the first colonial medical school, called for an end to such overlapping. "Just as generals do not dig trenches," he advised his colleagues in a lecture, "Discourse upon the Institution of Medical Schools in America," "so physicians need not perform the less dignified tasks of medical practice."9

Virtually no one in colonial days heeded Morgan's call. But they did accept the plea he made for formal education.

As early as 1647, John Eliot of Massachusetts had tried to get support from England to set up a medical school, but to little avail.10 Over the course of the colonial era, a few hundred wealthier men went abroad to study medicine, mainly in Edinburgh, Leyden, and London.

A few of these graduates returned home and offered public lectures and demonstrations for a fee. Students who completed this instruction were awarded certificates. Ultimately, in 1765, with Morgan's urging and the letters of recommendation Morgan had acquired from famous European physicians, the College of Pennsylvania agreed to open a department of medicine.

Dr. Morgan and Dr. William Shippen, both graduates of medical school in Edinburgh, Scotland, were invited to be the school's first faculty, and three more university-educated doctors were added. In 1768 the Philadelphia Medical School graduated its first class of ten students.

The same year, another medical school was founded in New York City at King's College, which later became Columbia University. After the Revolutionary War, which had interrupted medical education, two more schools—Harvard in 1782 and Dartmouth in 1797—were established.

By the time of the American Revolution, 400 of the colony's 3,500 doctors had a university education, and half of those 400 had earned a medical degree.11

Since there were no medical schools in the colonies

until 1765, and an education abroad was possible only for the wealthy, most men acquired medical training by apprenticing to a doctor.

For a year or more, the apprentice lived with his master and learned medicine by watching and assisting, and reading whatever medical books his master's library had. At first, his responsibilities were probably limited to grooming his master's horse and household chores. In time, he probably took on more medical duties, such as mixing medicine, cupping and bleeding, and assisting with amputations.[12]

Still other practitioners set up medical practices without ever apprenticing. They learned their trade from books like William Buchan's *Domestic Medicine*, Johan Blauber's *Chemistry*, Galen's *Art of Physics* and *The Unlearned Chemist*, or Philip Barrough's *Method of Physic*.[13] Or they learned from experience—through trial and error on their patients!

Few doctors let a lack of education stop them from practicing medicine. Indeed, in eighteenth-century Massachusetts, four out of five doctors had never attended medical school or even apprenticed to a doctor, compared to England where four out of five doctors apprenticed at least three years.[14]

To keep abreast of medical advances, some physicians read journals from Europe, particularly the *Transactions of the London Royal Society*. In 1762, Dr. John Morgan tried to raise colonial medical standards by starting an exclusive medical society similar to London's Royal College of Physicians.

According to Morgan's plan, the Philadelphia center would serve all the colonies by helping physicians exchange knowledge among themselves, encouraging research, and establishing and enforcing professional standards of conduct.[15]

Several state medical societies were established, but they were never on the scale that Morgan had envisioned. At the time, many colonists resisted anything that helped create trade monopolies. Thus, an atmosphere of fear that a powerful medical society would enable doctors to limit their medical services, charge excessive fees, and take advantage of their membership prevented the idea from taking root until the nineteenth century, when the American Medical Association was founded.

New York in 1760 and New Jersey in 1772 passed legislation requiring the examination and licensing of practicing physicians. Enforcing this new law, however, meant that patients would have to turn in the healers they engaged—an unlikely scenario. Consequently, the restrictions remained unenforced and ineffective for the rest of the colonial period.

Apparently, a lack of education stopped few physicians from practicing their trade. During the early colonial era, there was a shortage of doctors, particularly in sparsely populated areas. "The Virginians have but few Doctors among them," wrote John Oldmisor, of the scarcity there.[16]

As the colonial population grew, the number of healers increased. By the time the colonists sought freedom from England, there was one doctor for every six hundred people. Town populations boasted an even better ratio. In 1750, New York's ratio was 1:350, and in 1730, Williamsburg, Virginia, had a 1:135 ratio of doctors to residents.[17]

Unfortunately, even if doctors were available, most colonists were too poor to afford their fees. Lacking cash, colonists bartered corn, tobacco, and other products for medical care. In 1735, for example, Dr. Cornelius Van Dyck of Schenectady, New York, received tea, rum, sugar, and a cowhead. Another doctor in nearby Albany received ten beaver skins from one of his patients.[18]

Because few colonists could afford doctors' fees,

most doctors charged wealthier patients as much as possible in order to earn a living. Dr. William Douglass of Boston said that he could "live handsomely by the incomes of my Practice," and even claimed to have saved "some small matter."[19] Physicians less fortunate than Dr. Douglass had to rely on other sources of income. They turned to farming, public service, innkeeping, land speculation, and the ministry.

Given the shortage of doctors and their expensive fees, many people relied instead on home remedies. As a result, they were spared some of the more life-threatening treatments, such as excessive bloodletting, that were popular among prominent physicians.

Despite a brief apprenticeship and lack of formal education, American healers had an advantage over their sophisticated, better-educated European colleagues. For out of necessity, they often turned to simpler, and therefore safer, remedies.

Toward the end of the colonial period, a person could still practice medicine without a formal education or membership in a medical society, and most did. In time, though, it became possible for an aspiring doctor to get both formal training and professional membership—and homegrown at that.

## CHAPTER EIGHT

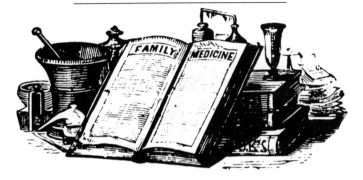

# In the Institutions

Today, most people are born in a hospital. When people are ill and injured, they go to hospitals or clinics. Included among these hospitals and clinics are some of the finest teaching hospitals, which have the world's highest medical standards. Compared to today's medical climate, colonial medicine had practically no standards—and hardly any hospitals.

The first known hospital in the British colonies was started in 1612 in Henricopolis, Virginia, a tiny settlement about fifty miles up the river from Jamestown, Virginia. Henricopolis failed to grow, and when its five inhabitants were killed by Native Americans ten years later, nothing remained of the hospital.

In 1620, the London Company, which had founded Jamestown, ordered construction of guest houses to "harbor sick men and receive strangers."[1] Again, though, little came of this plan. Once Virginia became a royal colony, nothing was heard about these guest houses again.

In 1658, the Dutch West India Company of New

Amsterdam, which later became New York, opened a hospital for its employees. This small institution was run by a woman named Hilletze Wilbruch under the direction of the company's physician. Like the other colonial hospitals of the era, it did not last long; twenty-two years after its founding it was abandoned.

As the colonies grew and permanent communities were established, some of the larger towns built almshouses where the poor could go. In these almshouses, or poorhouses as they were called, the homeless, the blind, orphans, the insane, and even criminals lived together. In some of the shelters, residents were expected to work for their room and board; such places became known as "workhouses."

During 1736 alone, two almshouses were founded in the British colonies—St. Philip's of Charleston and the Workhouse and House of Correction of New York City. A third, Charity House, was later founded in the French colonies.

Typically, an almshouse reserved a small room with a half-dozen or so beds for the sick. Sometimes a physician was assigned to treat patients, but usually fellow almshouse residents assumed responsibility for their care. Yet in these early almshouses, neither health care nor dignity had much meaning. For although shelter and food were offered, medical care was sporadic, and filthy, drafty, and overcrowded conditions prevailed.

Some of these almshouses and workhouses eventually became hospitals, but not until after the colonial era. Massachusetts General began as an almshouse,[2] as did Philadelphia General Hospital.[3]

Despite their ignorance of the causes of diseases, colonists had observed that diseases like smallpox were highly contagious. To isolate those who were infected from the rest of the population, and therefore prevent or minimize an epidemic, a few town and city governments established pesthouses, or lazar (leper) houses, as they were also called.

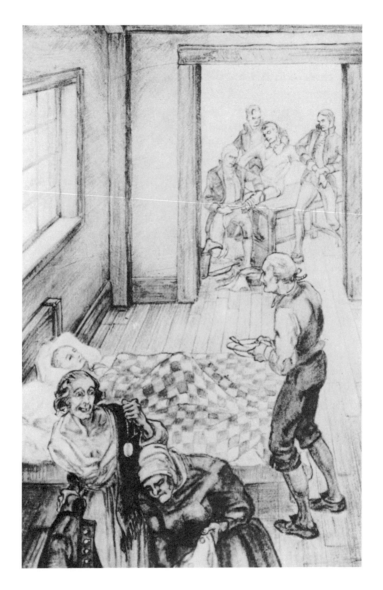

Colonial hospitals housed a melange of residents
that included homeless, the blind, orphans,
the insane, and even criminals. Moreover,
healthier patients were expected to help
with the housekeeping and other chores.

In 1717, the General Court of Massachusetts built pesthouses on Spectacle Island and Castle Williams to isolate infected sea passengers. In 1738, a pesthouse was erected on Bedloe's Island in New York Harbor for the same purpose. As late as the summer of 1794, during a scare of yellow fever, New York erected a pesthouse that eventually became Bellevue Hospital, one of New York's largest hospitals.[4]

Pesthouses harbored the same terrible conditions found in almshouses. Even worse perhaps, they offered no medical attention whatsoever. For their purpose was to protect the public from epidemic disease and not to treat the infected.

Fortunately, the majority of colonists were never condemned to live in either almshouses or pesthouses. They lived at home, most likely on a farm. Home was where they were born, where they stayed when sick or ailing, and where they probably died. If colonists were away from home, or didn't have one, they would probably go to someone else's, perhaps a doctor's home where his wife nursed a few of his patients.

The record of Virginia's Surrey Court describes how, in 1676, Dr. George Lee was "most reluctantly forced to take Mrs. Richard Hill into his house for medical care."[5] In Rappahannock County, Virginia, in 1686, James Stanford was granted 1,200 pounds of tobacco against the estate of Nathaniel Gubbs in "Recompence for his Care and the trouble of his house in the time of the Said Mr. Gubbs sickness."[6]

Although home was the mainstay of health care, a few individuals, primarily European-educated physicians, recognized the value of hospitals. Not only could hospitals help the poor sick to reenter society, the physicians reasoned that the experience in hospitals could also provide medical students with valuable clinical practice.

Writing in the *Pennsylvania Gazette*, Benjamin Franklin pointed out the economical advantages of hospital care. "Suppose a person is under the necessity of having a limb amputated," reasoned Franklin, "he must have the constant attendance of a nurse, a room, a fire, et cetera . . . which cannot be procured . . . at less expense than fifteen shillings a week. Whereas in a hospital, one nurse, one fire, et cetera . . . will be sufficient for ten patients."[7]

Franklin and his friend, Dr. Thomas Bond of Philadelphia, were so convincing that sufficient funds for a hospital were raised by the "public spirited inhabitants of Philadelphia," as the cornerstone declares. When Pennsylvania Hospital opened its doors in 1752, it became a model institution in the colonies and the earliest hospital still in use today.

For several reasons, Pennsylvania Hospital adopted a rather progressive policy. In contrast to almshouses where residents could live permanently, Pennsylvania admitted only patients who could be cured within a reasonable period (except for the insane, whom they housed in the basement). Furthermore, no one with an infectious disease was admitted unless that person could be isolated in a separate apartment. In addition, hospital policy prohibited mothers from keeping their children with them; children were considered too much of a burden to the hospital staff and "too noisesome to the other patients."[8]

To retain their self-respect and independence, Pennsylvania Hospital patients were expected to pay their own expenses. During the hospital's first eighty years, nearly half of the patients paid their own way.[9] Those who couldn't pay were admitted free, and if they were not too sick, they were given light housekeeping chores or simple nursing duties.

Private wards and rooms were available to anyone choosing to pay higher rates. But in the spirit of democracy, paying patients slept side-by-side with free patients.

Professors at King's College in New York City also

recognized the need for a hospital. Noting the success of Pennsylvania Hospital, three prominent physicians—Drs. Peter Middleton, John Jones, and Samuel Bard—lobbied for a similar institution. Just as Dr. Thomas Bond and Benjamin Franklin had raised private money to start Pennsylvania Hospital, the New York physicians raised private funds for their project. However, they also convinced the colonial legislature to subsidize their venture for twenty years.

*The Society of the Hospital of New York In America,* as the organization was called, faced major setbacks. First, a fire destroyed their original building. Then the Revolutionary War interfered with further development. Finally though, in January 1791, New York Hospital opened its doors to patients and joined with King's College to provide clinical experience for medical students. (Together, the hospital and medical school are now part of Columbia University.)

During the late 1700s, a movement to improve the treatment of the poor inspired a few of Philadelphia's wealthy patrons to start a dispensary (clinic) where the "indigent poor" could receive free treatment as outpatients (no overnight stays). In 1786, financed by annual membership dues, the Philadelphia Dispensary opened its doors, becoming the forerunner of emergency outpatient clinics.

Six physicians were appointed to serve the dispensary in two-month shifts without pay. The dispensary also staffed four consulting physicians, a surgeon, an apothecary, and a treasurer. Five years later, New Yorkers again followed Philadelphia's lead and started a similar institution.

Convinced that "kindness works better than brutality in treating mental illness," eighteenth-century Parisian Philippe Pinel removed the chains from fifty-three "lunaticks." His success with the experiment inspired reform in the treatment of the insane and mentally incompetent.[10]

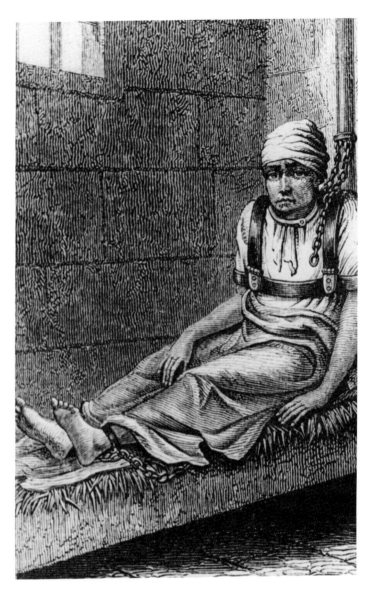

Mentally ill and insane patients received
harsh treatment. Even in hospitals, they
were confined to the basement and
restrained or shackled to their beds.

In response to this reform movement, Francis Fauquier, Virginia's royal governor, asked Virginia's House of Burgesses to fund a public mental hospital. Its purpose was to protect the populace from "those who are deprived of their sense and wander about the countryside terrifying the rest of their fellow creatures."[11] "These miserable Objects who cannot help themselves morally deserved to be treated," he argued, "in the hope that their 'lost reason' might be restored."[12]

At first, the House of Burgesses declined Fauquier's advice, but the governor persisted. When the Virginia legislature finally acquiesced, Eastern State Public Hospital of Williamsburg, Virginia, which opened in 1772, became the colonies' first mental hospital.

Compared to other mental wards of the time, Eastern State was remarkably successful. In its first ten years of operation, 20 percent of its patients were deemed cured and were discharged.

Despite such success, the insane were still frequently mistreated. For even at Eastern State, they were routinely given powerful drugs, bled, blistered, plunged into cold baths, and kept in mechanical restraints that did little to improve their condition, and most likely worsened it.

Undoubtedly, hospitals contributed to medical education. Because their conditions were so deplorable, however, colonial medical institutions could hardly be considered places of healing and care. In fact, as late as the nineteenth century, a stay in the hospital was considered to be "the last station on the way to the grave."[13]

## CHAPTER NINE

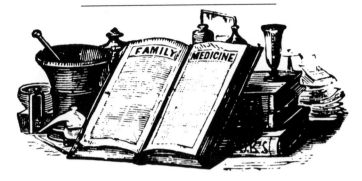

# Casualties of War

The Revolutionary War was fought with rifles, cannons, swords, and bayonets that killed, maimed, and wounded 1,000 Continental soldiers each year. Ironically, though, disease killed at least nine times as many soldiers.[1] "We lost not less than ten to twenty of camp disease," said Dr. James Tilton, a Delaware physician who later became Surgeon General of the Army, "for one by weapons of the enemy."[2]

Some 70,000 men died during the war.[3] Better food, clothing, hygiene, and medical care would have reduced that number and improved the lives of those who survived as well.

As men from the colonies mingled together in the camps, their germs mingled too, spreading typhus, smallpox, and influenza. Unsanitary conditions hosted more disease, such as typhoid and dysentery. Lack of food caused malnutrition and scurvy.

Conditions were so deplorable that Dr. Lewis Beeke, serving in the Canadian Campaign of 1776, doubted anyone would believe the horror. "No mortal

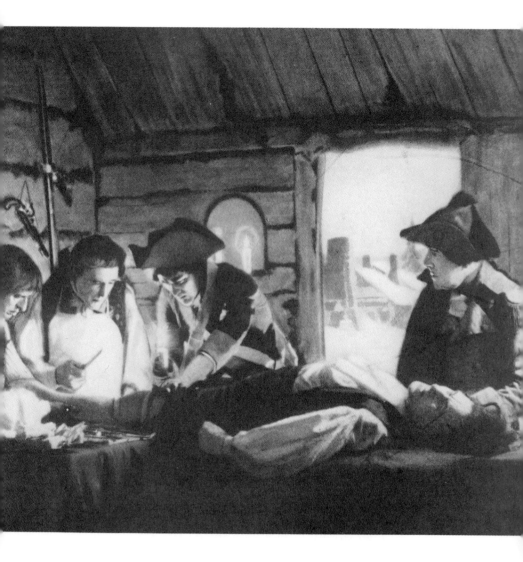

Lacking knowledge of antibiotics to fight infection, antiseptics to sterilize equipment, or even anesthesia to deaden the pain, Continental Army operations proved as dangerous to the soldiers as the battlefields.

will ever believe what these suffered unless they were eyewitnesses," he wrote. For Dr. Beeke saw men with inch-long maggots crawling out of their ears and "almost every part of the body."[4]

Even the weather invoked hardship. Soldiers suffered from exposure during the winter months and were ill-clad, ill-fed, and frequently sick. During the winter of 1777–78, Washington's troops endured bitter cold in damp, smoky log cabins, often going without shoes, shirts, food, or medicine. By the time the snow melted, nearly one-third of Washington's troops had perished from the ordeal.[5]

On the battlefield, hunger and disease weakened the men for fighting. In the camps, it demoralized them. Everywhere it lessened their chance of winning the war. "The men died so fast for some time," remarked Ebenezer Elmer, an army surgeon who tried transporting his sick by sled to where they could obtain better medical attention, "that the living grew wearied in digging graves."[6] In New York, just before the retreat across the Hudson to New Jersey, one out of three soldiers was too sick to fight. And in another movement, only half the men were well enough to fight.[7]

Armies need adequate food, supplies, and medical attention in the field and hospitals for the sick and wounded. As Dr. Benjamin Rush wrote in his pamphlet, *Directions for the Preserving of Health of Soldiers; Recommended to the Consideration of the Officers of the Army of the United States*, soldiers need adequate dress, diet, cleanliness, exercise, sanitation, and vegetables "necessary to proper diet." He warned that alcohol is injurious to health and should be avoided.[8]

Clearly, the Continental Army was found lacking in all these areas. It also lacked a clear chain of command. From the start, professional jealousy, incompetence, and political corruption bitterly divided the "Hospital for the Army," as the medical branch of the military was called.

On July 17, 1775, the Continental Congress established an army medical department to address the medical needs of an army that was estimated to consist of about twenty thousand men. It was to be headed by a director general, or a chief physician, who would be appointed by Congress at a salary of four dollars a day. The first physician Congress appointed to this position was Dr. Benjamin Church of Boston.

In addition to the chief physician, the army hired four surgeons, twenty surgeon's mates, an apothecary, a clerk, two storekeepers, and one nurse for every ten sick men.9

Furthermore, a plan was set up for two kinds of hospitals: general hospitals to be set up in relatively permanent locations, and temporary, or "flying," hospitals to be located near the actual battlefields.

From the start, the army medical department had problems. Although one-third of the doctors—about 1,200—served in the army at one time or another, there was always a shortage of trained medical personnel. Furthermore, both Congress and the provincial governments in each colony had failed to provide sufficient funds, equipment, or supplies. Finally, corruption among those responsible for distributing supplies prevented many soldiers and units from being adequately equipped.

Rivalries between the medical directors eroded the chain of command, as Drs. John Morgan and William Shippen, Jr., once friends, now feuded and became bitter enemies. For a while, Dr. Shippen became director of the army department, but like Dr. Morgan, he, too, was asked to resign over a dispute.

Until the war was well along, even George Washington failed to grasp the importance of a healthy army. As late as January 1777, Washington marched his troops from Trenton to Princeton without taking along a single surgeon or warning his medical officers of the move.

When Washington did try to raise the medical standards by requiring surgeons and their mates to pass an examination, he met with disapproval. Few states complied with his request, and New Jersey went so far as to formally reject a bill establishing an examining board.[10]

Wherever room could be found—in barns, private homes, soldiers' huts, and churches—the general hospitals were established. Or they were built especially for the army. However, these hospitals lacked everything from beds, medicine, and food to blankets and straw for the mattresses.

At first, bedding straw in these facilities was rarely changed and troops were crowded closely together. These conditions spread disease. By the end of the war, the importance of hygiene, fresh air, and exercise was recognized. With improved conditions came improved health.

As we already learned, typhus is carried by bed and body lice, and typhoid and dysentery are spread through contaminated food and drink. These diseases wore down the men's resistance, giving them a variety of symptoms that included chronic diarrhea, fevers, skin eruptions, deliriums, severe headaches, and a dry, black, crusty tongue.

By learning to air their blankets each day and burn the straw of previous patients, typhus (which was so widespread it was called hospital or jail fever) and dysentery were cut down. Other measures taken, such as providing more room for patients, and circulating fresh air, also improved the situation somewhat.

Many of the troops came from isolated areas of the country where they had never been exposed to smallpox, and therefore lacked immunity against it. Consequently, when they were exposed to smallpox in the camps, it took a tremendous toll of lives. In response to the problem, in 1777, Washington initiated a widespread inoculation program that dramatically improved the situation.

Dysentery constantly sapped the soldiers' strength. Amoebae and bacteria were found in contaminated, spoiled food and drink, and were further spread by human waste and filth, which accompanied soldiers wherever they went.

Many soldiers suffered from "bilious fever." Jaundiced and vomiting, or excreting blood, they were also victimized by the "itch," malaria, venereal disease, rheumatism, pleurisy, and simple nostalgia. Homesickness, as Dr. James Thacher explained, caused "perplexing instances or indisposition occasioned by absence from home."[11] His remedy was simple: "The only expedient . . . effectual for their relief is to billet them in the country, where they can enjoy pure air and a milk diet, or to furlough them to their homes, if within reach."[12]

Even though disease and famine affected more lives, battles certainly did cause their share of damage. When fired at close range, the large round musket balls caused gunshot wounds of brutal damage. If the ball was imbedded less than "a finger's length" in the flesh, it was removed with a special spoon-shaped forcep. If it was deeper, however, it was left in place.

When Native Americans fought, their tomahawks and knives inflicted cuts that had to be closed with stitches, bandages, and sticking plasters.

Compound fractures of the joints and shattered bones necessitated amputation, which required sharp instruments and considerable skill in order to prevent too much blood loss. Infection was so common, though, that it inspired the grim joke: "The operation was a success but the patient died."

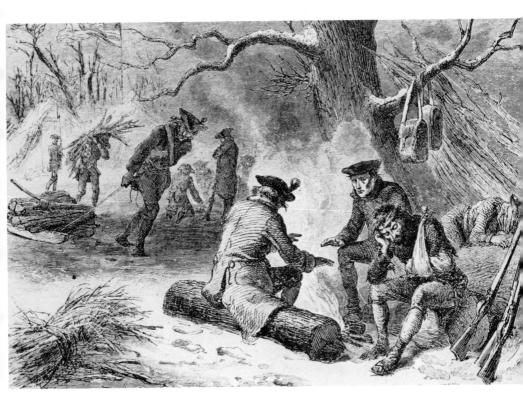

Battle wounds were common, but
starvation, malnutrition, and
disease claimed *nine times* more
lives among Continental troops.

Each year of the war, approximately 10,000 soldiers died.[13] Yet despite so many deaths on and off the
battlefield, Americans won the war—against a better-
trained, better-equipped enemy. Tragically, though,
with better sanitation and medical leadership, many
of those men might have survived to experience the
victory.

## CHAPTER TEN

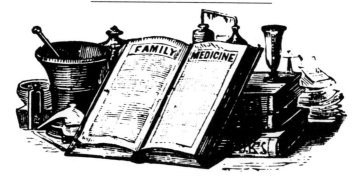

# Staying Healthy

"**P**revention is the better cure, so says the proverb and 'tis sure," advised Nathaniel Cotton in his book, *Vision in Verse*, published in 1751.[1] Considering the cures of the day—from blistering and bleeding to heroic medicines and gruesome amputations—no doubt many colonists tried to heed such advice and maintain whatever health they had.

In time, colonists learned the value of a diet that includes fresh fruit and vegetables. In time, they learned the value of fresh air, exercise, and adequate rest. And although they did not know the exact reason why certain diseases came from swampy, low-lying marshes or filthy, poorly drained land, in time, they tried to clean up such areas.

For two cool evenings in March 1779, the Drinker's cesspool, located in the backyard behind their lovely Philadelphia home, was cleaned. "Five men with two Carts & c. are about a dirty Jobb in our Yard to night," wrote Elizabeth Drinker. "They are removing the offering from ye temple of Cloaciina."[2] It was the first time the Drinker's cesspool had been cleaned in forty-four years.

Other colonists cleaned their own privies. But unlike the Drinker's, who had the contents carted off, they dumped their waste directly into the street. Twenty years after her cesspool was first cleaned, Elizabeth Drinker detected other people cleaning theirs—from the foul smell in the air. "There has been more work of that sort done this Winter in this City," she remarked in her diary, "than ever was . . . in any winter before, or perhaps in any to come."[3]

From their lack of personal hygiene to their lack of public sanitation, colonists were never noted for cleanliness. Because colonists believed that soap and water washed away oils protecting them from "miasma" and "bad vapors" that can enter the body through the skin's pores and other openings, they avoided bathing.

Elizabeth Drinker was rather progressive when she showered for the first time—as an adult. "I bore it better than I expected," she wrote of her experience, "not having been wett all over at once for twenty-eight years."[4]

Often the sight of garbage, rubbish, and dead animals on colonial streets was particularly loathsome. Some towns hired scavengers to get rid of the debris. Other towns fined those who put garbage in the street in the first place, such as butchers who discarded offal and bones.

For the most part, individuals were responsible for keeping the streets in front of their homes clean. Frequently though, drains and open street sewers became receptacles for every type of debris that eventually drained into the harbor slips. Unbearable odors rose from the open sewage and rotting garbage, particularly in the summer months when the tide was low and the matter was exposed to the air.

As we have already learned, colonial water supplies

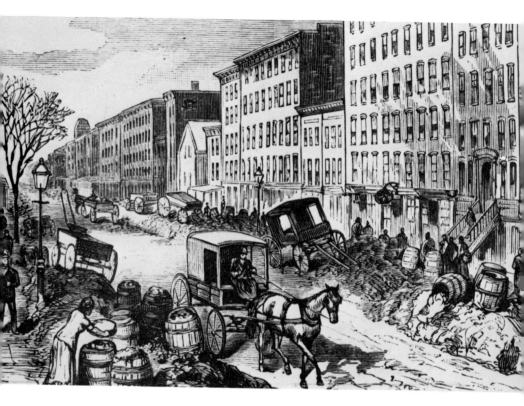

Even after colonial days, city streets filled
up with offal and other garbage. In addition,
nearby swamps bred malarial and yellow
fever-carrying mosquitoes. Such deplorable
lack of sanitation brought widespread disease.

were never sanitary. Moreover, lacking knowledge of
germs, no one boiled water to make it sanitary. Yet
without such sanitation, colonists picked up dysentery,
typhoid, and other ailments from the water supply.
When larger wells were dug to serve several families or
an entire village, such disease spread all the more.

If the well water was unappealing because it was too brackish, for example, as much of the well water was inclined to be, many colonists turned to alternatives. Sometimes they had fresh spring water delivered. In 1761, New York licensed spring water carriers. But even if the spring water tasted superior and looked cleaner, it could still harbor disease.

Another alternative to drinking well water was drinking hard liquor. Even children and babies were given such beverages. By 1830, the average American was guzzling seven gallons of hard liquor per year.[5]

Alcohol and liquor presented health problems beyond addiction and liver damage. If they were distilled in lead pipes, as eighteenth-century rum and cider were apt to be, they could cause lead poisoning. Eventually, physicians recognized that the "dry belly-ake" associated with rum and English cider was caused by lead poisoning. To alleviate the problem, Massachusetts passed legislation in 1728 that prevented the distillation of alcoholic beverages in lead pipes.

Despite a few sanitation measures, there was still little the colonists knew about prevention, but they thought they knew a lot. To avoid breathing "miasma" and "catching" diseases such as smallpox or yellow fever from the air, they held vinegar-soaked rags over their noses, wore amulets of animal teeth or bags of camphor around their necks, or carried lengths of tarred rope.

Those who could, locked themselves indoors and chewed garlic or wore it in their shoes. When a rumor spread that gunpowder might deter disease, "Philadelphians shot at the miasma from their windows until so many were wounded the mayor forbade it."[6]

Amid such folklore and spotty methods of prevention, there was one bright spot in colonial medical history—inoculation against smallpox.

Throughout the colonial period, recurring smallpox epidemics were among the most feared and deadly. Noting the connection between contact with a smallpox patient and the spread of the disease, some towns enacted quarantines to isolate infected patients. Unfortunately, quarantine laws were often ignored, or enacted too long after the disease had started spreading.

In April 1721, smallpox threatened Boston and the surrounding area. Around that time, Reverend Cotton Mather had learned about a procedure used in the Middle East and in parts of Africa.

Pus from a blister of a person with an active case of smallpox was placed in a small incision on the arm of a healthy person. Although the person would get smallpox, it was usually limited to a mild case, from which the patient normally recovered. Afterward, the person was immune to the disease. (While the person had it, however, he or she was highly contagious, a fact many people ignored, thus spreading the disease to others.)

Because people *could* die from inoculation, criticism of the procedure was strong. In Boston, criticism came from such eminent physicians as Dr. William Douglass, the city's only medical school graduate. Public outcry against Reverend Mather was so great, in fact, that someone even threw a bomb into his window, with the following note: "Cotton Mather, you dog; Damn you: I'll inoculate you with this, with a pox to you."[7]

Amid this atmosphere of protest, Mather kept up his campaign to convince the medical community of the benefits of inoculation. Although he had support

One of the most significant medical discoveries of the colonial era is the smallpox inoculation, which led the way to the safer cowpox inoculation discovered by Edward Jenner in 1897.

# AN
## Hiſtorical ACCOUNT
### OF THE
# SMALL-POX
## INOCULATED
### IN
## NEW ENGLAND,

Upon all Sorts of Perſons, *Whites*, *Blacks*, and of all Ages and Conſtitutions.

With ſome Account of the Nature of the Infection in the NATURAL and INOCULATED Way, and their different Effects on HUMAN BODIES.

With ſome ſhort DIRECTIONS to the UN-EXPERIENCED in this Method of Practice.

Humbly dedicated to her Royal Highneſs the Princeſs of WALES,
## By *Zabdiel Boylſton*, F. R. S.

*The Second Edition,* Corrected.

### LONDON:

Printed for S. CHANDLER, at the Croſs-Keys in the *Poultry.*
M. DCC. XXVI.

Re-Printed at BOSTON in N. E. for S. GERRISH in *Cornhil,* and T. HANCOCK at the Bible and Three Crowns in *Annſtreet.* M. DCC. XXX.

from many of his fellow clergy, most doctors remained opposed to the procedure.

Then, Dr. Zabdiel Boylston received a persuasive letter from Reverend Mather. Boylston decided not only to inoculate patients, but to publicize his undertaking in the newspaper. Despite continued pressure on him to suspend his experiment, Boylston inoculated some 240 patients, including his own and Mather's children. Another forty people were inoculated by a few other doctors.

The epidemic lasted a year. Nearly half of Boston's populace came down with smallpox. Of those infected, 844 people, or about 15 percent, died. Only six of those who were inoculated—about 2 percent—died, confirming the success of the procedure.[8]

Eventually, both doctors and the public became convinced of the value of inoculation. For in town after town, the percentage of those who died from inoculation versus those who died from contracting the disease was significantly less.

By the time of Philadelphia's 1753 epidemic, inoculation was such a proven health measure that Benjamin Franklin urged everyone to practice it. Citing the advantages of inoculation, he was sure that even if the chance were "*two* to *one* in favour of the practice among children . . . surely parents will no longer refuse to accept the practice."[9]

In 1796, the British physician Edward Jenner announced his discovery of the cowpox vaccine, a far safer alternative to inoculation (because it uses a milder strain of the pox virus). Unlike inoculation, vaccination was widely accepted from the start.

Together, inoculation and vaccination against smallpox became one of the most important medical discoveries of colonial times—if not the only one, however. For even at the end of the colonial era, medicine still had a long way to go. A very long way indeed.

# Significant Beginnings

**1607** Jamestown was founded, beginning English colonization

**1610** Lawrence Bohun, the first doctor in the English colonies, arrived

**1616** Smallpox epidemic in New England nearly destroys the Native American tribes from the Penobscot River to Narragansett Bay

**1721** First inoculation against smallpox in the colonies took place

**1735** First diphtheria epidemic in New England began

**1750** First human dissection was performed by Drs. John Bard and Peter Middleton of New York City on the body of Hermannus Carrol, an executed murderer

**1765** First department of medicine in the colonies started by Drs. John Morgan and William Shippen at the College of Philadelphia

**1775** Dr. Benjamin Church appointed the first surgeon general of the Continental Army

**1785** First dispensary was established in Philadelphia by Dr. Benjamin Rush

**1790** First census was taken in the United States

**1797** First medical periodical in the United States, called *The Medical Repository*, was published

**1798** First attempt at formal nursing instruction

**1798** Dr. Edward Jenner discovers a vaccination against smallpox

# Source Notes

## CHAPTER ONE

**1.** David Freeman Hawke, *The Colonial Experience* (New York: Bobbs-Merrill, 1966), 82.

**2.** Quoted in Gary Frances Dow, *Everyday Life in the Massachusetts Bay Colony* (New York: Benjamin Bloom, 1937, reprinted 1967), 175–6.

## CHAPTER TWO

**1.** Quoted in Milton Meltzer, *The American Revolutionaries* (New York: Thomas Y. Crowell, 1987), 7.

**2.** Ibid., 8.

**3.** Hawke, *Everyday Life in Early America* (New York: Harper & Row, 1988), 72.

**4.** Quoted in John B. Blake, "Diseases and Medical Practice in Colonial America," *History of American Medicine: A Symposium*, Felix Marti-Ibanez, ed. (New York: MD Publications, 1958), 34.

**5.** Quoted in Wyndham Blanton, *Medicine in Virginia in the Seventeenth Century* (Richmond, Va.: William Byrd Press, 1930), 43.

**6.** Quoted in Henry E. Sigerist, *American Medicine*, translated by Hildegard Nagel (New York: W.W. Norton & Co., 1934), 31.

**7.** Quoted in Blanton, *Medicine in Virginia*, 42.

**8.** James Cassedy, *Demography in Early America* (Cambridge, Mass.: Harvard University, 1969), 24.

**9.** John Duffy, *Epidemics in Colonial America* (Baton Rouge, La.: Louisiana State University, 1953), 13.

**10.** Robert I. Groler, *The Healing Arts in America*, pamphlet, (New York: Fraunces Tavern Museum, 1985), 17.

**11.** Blanton, *Medicine in Virginia*, 60.

**12.** Duffy, private correspondence with author, 9 September 1991.

**13.** Colonel P. M. Ashburn, *The Ranks of Death* (New York: Coward-McCann, 1947), 32.

**14.** The majority of slaves actually arrived in the seventeenth century.

**15.** Estimates vary between 15 percent to about 30 percent on slave ships. In "Slavery in America," *African American*, 5th ed., Harry A. Ploski and James Wilhams, eds. (Detroit: Gale Research, 1989), 1433.

**16.** Ibid.

**17.** Todd L. Savitt, *Fevers, Agues and Cures: Medical Life in Old Virginia*, pamphlet (Richmond, Va.: Virginia Historical Society, 1991), 19.

**18.** Helen Brock, "North America, A Western Outpost of European Medicine," *The Medical Enlightenment of the Eighteenth Century*, Andrew Cunningham and Roger French, eds. (New York: Cambridge University Press, 1990), 214.

**19.** Ibid., 211.

**20.** Cassedy, *Demography in Early America*, pp. 14–5; Duffy, *Epidemics*, 13–4.

**21.** Blake, "Diseases and Medical Practice in Colonial America, 35.

---

**22.** Duffy, *Epidemics*, 15.

**23.** This figure is only an estimate for the original English colonies. It does not include all of the thirteen colonies since many came into existence after 1700. Duffy, private correspondence, 9 September 1991; also cited in Erick H. Christianson, "Medicine in New England," *Medicine in the New World*, Ronald L. Numbers, ed. (Knoxville, Tenn.: University of Tennessee, 1987), 112.

## CHAPTER THREE

**1.** Duffy, *Epidemics*, 170.

**2.** Cecil K. Drinker, *Not So Long Ago* (New York: Oxford University Press, 1937), 108.

**3.** Duffy, *Epidemics*, 170.

**4.** Quoted in Ibid., 78.

**5.** Ibid., 80.

**6.** John Duffy, *The Sanitarians* (Urbana and Chicago: University of Illinois, 1990), 10.

**7.** Duffy, *Epidemics*, 41.

**8.** Peter H. Wood, "The Impact of Smallpox on the Native American Population," *Early American Medicine* (New York: Fraunces Tavern Museum, 1987), 26–8.

**9.** J. Adair, *History of the American Indians*, 1775, reprinted 1966 (Ann Arbor: University of Michigan Press), 27.

**10.** Duffy, *Epidemics*, 239.

**11.** Drinker, *Not So Long Ago*, 127.

**12.** Ibid., 67–90.

**13.** Richard Harrison Shyrock, *Medicine and Society in America: 1660–1860* (Ithaca, N.Y.: Cornell University, 1960), 92.

**14.** Laurel Thatcher Ulrich, *A Midwife's Tale* (New York: Alfred A. Knopf, 1990), 170.

**15.** Duffy, *Epidemics*, 7; Leonard Everett Fisher, *The Hospitals* (New York: Holiday House, 1980), 12.

**16.** Frank Kendig and Richard Hutton, *Lifespans* (New York: Holt, Rinehart & Winston, 1979), 8; Forty percent of infants died, according to Oscar Theodore Barck, Jr. and Hugh Talmage Lefler, *Colonial America* (New York: Macmillan, 1958), 425.

**17.** Drinker, *Not So Long Ago*, 110.

**18.** Barck and Lefler, *Colonial America*, 426.

**19.** Duffy, *Epidemics*, 240.

**20.** Blake, "Diseases and Medical Practice," 38–9.

**21.** Hawke, *Everyday Life in Early America*, 72.

**22.** The average life expectancy in sixty Massachusetts and New Hampshire communities in 1789 was 34.5 years for men and 36.5 years for women. Cited in Groler, *The Healing Arts in America*, 39.

**23.** In Andover, Massachusetts, twenty-year-old males had a life expectancy of sixty-five years, whereas females had one of sixty-two. In contrast, in Middlesex, Virginia, twenty-year-old males had a life expectancy of forty-nine years, and females only forty. Furthermore, 50 percent of women and 60 percent of all colonial men lived to be fifty; 30 percent of the total population lived to be seventy. Hawkes, *The Colonial Experience*, 73, and Shyrock, *Medicine and Society*, 108.

**24.** Cassedy, *Demography in Early America*, 265.

**25.** Ibid.

**26.** Quoted in Cassedy, *Demography in Early America*, 265.

**27.** Quoted in Ibid., 264.

**28.** Blake, "Diseases and Medical Practice," 38.

## CHAPTER FOUR

**1.** Margaret M. Coffin, *Death in Early America* (New York: Thomas Nelson, 1976), 188–9.

**2.** Ibid., 187.

**3.** Martin Kaufman, *American Medical Education* (Westport, CT.: Greenwood Press, 1976), 31.

**4.** David L. Cowen, *Medicine and Health in New Jersey* (Princeton, N.J.: D. Van Nostrand, 1964), 7.

**5.** Duffy, *Epidemics*, 6.

**6.** Quoted in William Frederick Norwood, "Medicine in the Era of the American Revolution," *History of American Medicine: A Symposium* (New York: M.D. Publications, 1959), 67.

**7.** Savitt, *Fevers, Agues and Cures*, 8.

**8.** Ibid., 10.

**9.** Sherwin Nuland, *Doctors: The Biography of Medicine* (New York: Alfred Knopf, 1988), 147.

## CHAPTER FIVE

**1.** Dow, *Everyday Life*, 190.

**2.** James Thomas Flexner, *Doctors on Horseback* (New York: Dover, 1957), 34.

**3.** Duffy, *Epidemics*, 95.

**4.** Flexner, *Doctors on Horseback*, 94.

**5.** Drinker, *Not So Long Ago*, 126.

**6.** Duffy, *The Healers*, 96.

**7.** Drinker, *Not So Long Ago*, 107–8.

**8.** Dow, *Everyday Life*, 175.

**9.** Cowen, *Medicine and Health in New Jersey*, 29.

**10.** Ibid.

**11.** Drinker, *Not So Long Ago*, 45.

**12.** Groler, *The Healing Arts in America*, 41.

## CHAPTER SIX

**1.** Dow, *Everyday Life*, 188.

**2.** Coffin, *Death in Early America*, 25.

**3.** J. Worth Estes, "Patterns of Drug Use in Early America," *Early American Medicine*, pamphlet (New York: Fraunces Tavern Museum, 1988), 33.

**4.** Ulrich, *A Midwife's Tale*, 50.

**5.** Bobbie Kalman, *Early Health and Medicine* (New York: Crabtree Publishing, 1983), 11.

**6.** Richard Le Strange, *A History of Herbal Plants* (New York: Arco, 1977), xvii.

**7.** Savitt, *Fevers, Agues and Cures*, 13.

**8.** Blanton, *Medicine in Virginia*, 109–11.

**9.** Groler, *Healing Arts in America*, 16.

**10.** Blanton, *Medicine in Virginia*, 111.

**11.** Ulrich, *A Midwife's Tale*, 50–1.

**12.** John Duffy, *The Healers* (New York: McGraw-Hill, 1976), 29.

**13.** Blanton, *Medicine in Virginia*, 108.

**14.** Kalman, *Early Health and Medicine*, 16.

**15.** Quoted in David Courtwright, *Dark Paradise: Opiate Addiction in America before 1940* (Cambridge, Mass.: Harvard University Press, 1982), 43.

**16.** Ibid.

**17.** Cowen, *Medicine and Health in New Jersey*, 28.

**18.** Estes, "Patterns of Drug Use," 35.

## CHAPTER SEVEN

**1.** Coffin, *Death in Early America*, 43.

**2.** Ibid.

**3.** Quoted in Beck, "Medicine in the Colonies," 34.

**4.** William Dosite Postell, "Medical Education and Medical Schools in Colonial America," *History of Medicine*, Felix Marti-Ibanez, ed. (New York: MD Publications, 1958), 48.

**5.** Henry R. Viets, M.D., *A Brief History of Medicine in Massachusetts* (Boston and New York: Houghton Mifflin Co., 1930), 28–34.

**6.** Ulrich, *A Midwife's Tale*, 63–4.

**7.** Kate Campbell-Hurd, *Women in Medicine* (Haddam, CT.: Haddam Press, 1938), 441.

**8.** Postell, 50.

**9.** Paraphrased in Shyrock, *Medicine and Society in America: 1660–1860*, 26.

**10.** Blake, *Public Health in the Town of Boston* (Cambridge, Mass.: Harvard University, 1959), 190.

**11.** Sigerist, *American Medicine*, 40–1.

**12.** Ibid., 33.

**13.** Hawke, *The Colonial Experience*, 300; Brock, "North America," 201.

**14.** Brock, "North America," 196–7.

**15.** Ibid., 203–4.

**16.** Duffy, *Sanitarians*, 16.

**17.** Shyrock, *Medicine and Society in America*, 12.

**18.** Coffin, *Death in Early America*, 34.

**19.** Quoted in Blake, *Public Health in the Town of Boston*, 198.

## CHAPTER EIGHT

**1.** Blanton, *History of Virginia*, 150.

**2.** Sigerist, *American Medicine*, 206.

**3.** Duffy, *The Healers*, 56.

**4.** Sigerist, *American Medicine*, 205–6.

**5.** Ibid.

**6.** Ibid., 157.

**7.** Mary Risley, *The House of Healing* (New York: Doubleday, 1961), 216.

**8.** Duffy, *The Healers*, 58.

**9.** Risley, *The House of Healing*, 216.

**10.** George Rosen, "Hospital," *Encyclopedia Americana*, vol. 14 (Danbury, CT.: Grolier, Inc., 1990), 347–43.

**11.** Shomer S. Zwelling, "Inside the Public Hospital," *Journal of Colonial Williamsburg Foundation* (Spring 1985), 21–4.

**12.** Ibid.

**13.** Risley, *The House of Healing* (New York: Doubleday, 1961), 208.

## CHAPTER NINE

**1.** William Frederick Norwood, "Medicine in the Era of the American Revolution," *History of American Medicine: A Symposium*, Felix Marti-Ibanez, ed. (New York: MD Publications, 1959), 63.

**2.** Quotes in Duffy, *The Healers*, 77.

**3.** Norwood, "Medicine in the Era of the American Revolution," 63.

**4.** Quoted in Meltzer, *American Revolutionaries*, 140–141.

**5.** Ira D. Gruber, "Valley Forge," *Encyclopedia Americana*, vol. 27 (Danbury, Conn.: Grolier Inc., 1990), 865.

**6.** David L. Cowen, *Medicine in Revolutionary New Jersey*, pamphlet (Trenton, N.J.: New Jersey Historical Commission, 1975), 10.

**7.** Cowen, *Medicine in New Jersey*, 25.

**8.** Ibid., 33.

**9.** Duffy, *The Healers*, 80.

**10.** Cowen, *Medicine in Revolutionary New Jersey*, 11.

**11.** Ibid., 24.

**12.** Quoted in Duffy, *The Healers*, 29.

**13.** Ibid., 77.

## CHAPTER TEN

**1.** Nathaniel Cotton, *Vision in Verse* (1751).

**2.** Drinker, *Not So Long Ago*, 26.

**3.** Ibid., 27.

**4.** Quoted in Drinker, *Not So Long Ago*, 28.

**5.** Arnold Trebach, cited in Congressional hearings on drugs (29 September 1988).

**6.** Coffin, *Death in Early America*, 18.

**7.** Duffy, *Epidemics in Colonial America*, 245.

**8.** Hawke, *The Colonial Experience*, 101.

**9.** Cassedy, *Demography in Early America*, 134–5.

# Glossary

**Ague**—chills

**Almshouse**—poorhouse

**Anesthetic**—something that causes a patient to feel less pain or no pain during surgery

**Apothecary**—a druggist or pharmacist; also a drugstore during the colonial era

**Apprentice**—a person who enters a legal agreement to work for a certain length of time with someone who can teach him or her a craft or trade, in order to learn that craft or trade

**Benefit**—herbs used to prevent illness or disease

**Blister**—to burn the skin until it forms sores (swellings that contain a liquid); in colonial times, blistering was done to "draw out a disease"

**Calenture**—term for yellow fever, a disease causing high fever and blood-filled vomit

**Calomel**—a medicine whose main ingredient is mercury chloride

**Cathartic**—a medicine causing person to have a bowel movement; laxative

**Consumption**—respiratory illness that persisted and "wasted away" the patient's health

**Distemper, throat**—diphtheria or scarlet fever

**Dropsy**—colonial term to describe too much fluid in the body

**Emetic**—medicine that causes people to vomit

**Endemic**—diseases that are always around

**Epidemic**—the rapid spread of a contagious disease among many people

**Flux**—old-fashioned term for any intestinal disorder, such as diarrhea or dysentery

**Gruel**—thin, liquid food made by boiling cereal in milk or water

**Infection**—a disease caused by germs or viruses

**Infectious**—spread by infection

**Inoculate**—to put a special form of the germs of a disease into a person's body to prevent or cure that disease

**Lancet**—a sharp instrument used to cut a vein for bleeding

**Miasma**—heavy vapor rising from the earth, once thought to cause disease

**Midwife**—a person skilled in helping women with childbirth; most midwives are female

**Phlebotomy**—bleeding a patient to reduce a fever or to treat other symptoms

**Poultice**—moist, hot mass of flour or mustard applied to sore part of the body

**Privy**—outdoor toilet

**Purge**—causing a person to empty the bowels

**Quarantine**—isolating someone in order to prevent the spreading of a contagious disease

**Scarlet fever**—contagious disease marked by bright red rash, high fever, and sore throat

**Simple**—herbs that are supposed to cure an illness or disease

**Tracheotomy**—cutting open the throat to help a patient breathe

**Typhoid fever**—fever caused by bacteria in bad water and food and marked by reddish spots on the skin and inflammation of the intestines

**Vaccine**—weak or dead germs of a disease that are prepared and injected as protection against that disease

**Vascular tension**—tension that colonists thought was caused by too much blood in the vein

**Vermin**—insects and other bugs

# Bibliography

Barck, Jr., Oscar Theodore, and Hugh Talmage Lefler. 1958. *Colonial America*. New York: Macmillan.

Beck, John B., M.D. 1966. *Medicine in the American Colonies*. Albuquerque, N.M.: Horn & Wallace.

Blake, John. 1959. *Public Health in the Town of Boston*. Cambridge, Mass.: Harvard University.

Blanton, Wyndham B. 1930. *Medicine in Virginia in the Seventeenth Century*. Richmond, Va.: William Byrd Press.

Boorstin, Daniel J. 1958. *The Americans: The Colonial Experience*. New York: Random House.

Cassedy, James H. 1969. *Demography in Early America*. Cambridge, Mass.: Harvard University.

Coffin, Margaret M. 1976. *Death in Early America*. New York: Thomas Nelson.

Cowen, David L. 1964. *Medicine and Health in New Jersey: A History*. Princeton, N.J.: D. Van Nostrand Co.

————. 1975. *Medicine in Revolutionary New Jersey*. pamphlet. Trenton, N.J.: New Jersey Historical Commission.

Cunningham, Andrew, and Roger French, eds. 1990. *The Medical Enlightenment of the Eighteenth Century.* New York: Cambridge University Press.

Dow, Gary Frances. 1935, reprinted 1967. *Everyday Life in the Massachusetts Bay Colony.* New York: Benjamin Bloom.

Drinker, Cecil K. 1937. *Not So Long Ago: A Chronicle of Medicine and Doctors in Colonial Philadelphia.* New York: Oxford University Press.

Duffy, John. 1953. *Epidemics in Colonial America.* Baton Rouge, La.: Louisiana State University Press.

————. 1976. *The Healers: The Rise of the Medical Establishment.* New York: McGraw-Hill.

————. 1990. *The Sanitarians: A History of American Public Health.* Urbana and Chicago: University of Illinois.

Fisher, Leonard Everett. 1980. *The Hospitals.* New York: Holiday House.

Flexner, James Thomas. 1957, reprinted 1969. *Doctors on Horseback: Pioneers of American Medicine.* New York: Dover Publications.

Hawke, David. 1966. *The Colonial Experience.* New York: Bobbs-Merrill.

Hughes, Thomas P. 1957. *Medicine in Virginia, 1607–1699.* pamphlet. Williamsburg, Va.: Virginia 350th Anniversary Celebration Corporation.

Kalman, Bobbie. 1983. *Early Health and Medicine.* New York: Crabtree Publishing.

Kaufman, Martin. 1976. *American Medical Education: The Formative Years, 1765–1910.* Westport, Conn.: Greenwood Press.

Marti-Ibanez, Felix, M.D., ed. 1959. *History of American Medicine: A Symposium.* no. 5. New York: MD Publications.

Mather, Cotton. reprinted 1972. *The Angel of Bethesda.* Barre, Mass.: American Antiquarian Society and Barre Publishers.

Packard, Francis R., M.D. 1931, reprinted 1963. *History of Medicine in the United States.* Vols. 1, 2. New York: Hafner Publishing.

Savitt, Todd L. 1991. *Fevers, Agues and Cures: Medical Life in Old Virginia.* pamphlet. Richmond, Va.: Virginia Historical Society.

Shyrock, Richard Harrison. 1960. *Medicine and Society in America: 1660–1860.* Ithaca, N. Y.: Cornell University Press.

Sigerist, Henry E., M.D. 1934. *American Medicine.* Translated by Hildegard Nagel. New York: W.W. Norton & Co.

Ulrich, Laurel Thatcher. 1990. *A Midwife's Tale: The Life of Martha Ballard, Based on Her Diary, 1785–1812.* New York: Alfred A. Knopf.

Viets, Henry R., M.D. 1930. *A Brief History of Medicine in Massachusetts.* Boston: Houghton Mifflin Company.

Vogel, Virgil J. 1970. *American Indian Medicine.* Norman, Okla.: University of Oklahoma Press.

Waring, Joseph Ioor, M.D. 1964. *A History of Medicine in South Carolina 1670–1825.* Charleston: South Carolina Medical Association.

Wesley, John. 1747, reprinted 1960. *Primitive Physic.* London: The Epworth Press.

See also: *Bulletin of the History of Medicine* and *Journal of the History of Medicine* found in medical libraries.

# Index

# About the Author

Susan Neiburg Terkel is the author of several books for young people, including *Understanding Child Custody, Should Drugs Be Legalized?*, and *Abortion: Facing the Issues*. Ms. Terkel lives in Hudson, Ohio, with her husband and three children.

94-274

12539-4

362.1     Terkel, Susan Neiburg
TER          Colonial American
                medicine

13.30